Assessing Financing, Education, Management and Policy Context for Strategic Planning of Human Resources for Health

Thomas Bossert | Till Bärnighausen | Diana Bowser
Andrew Mitchell | Gülin Gedik

World Health Organization

WHO Library Cataloguing-in-Publication Data

Assessing financing, education, management and policy context for strategic planning of human resources for health / Thomas Bossert [… et al.].

1.Health manpower- economics. 2.Health personnel - education. 3.Health manpower - organization and administration. 4.Public policy. 5.Strategic planning. 6.Decison making. 7.Motivation. I.World Health Organization. II.Bossert, Thomas.

ISBN 978 92 4 154731 4   (NLM classification: W 76)

Table of Contents

ACRONYMS AND ABBREVIATIONS

AIDS   Acquired Immunodeficiency Syndrome
DFID   United Kingdom Department for International Development
GDP   Gross Domestic Product
HRD   Human Resources Development
HRH   Human Resources for Health
HRM   Human Resources Management
ILO   International Labour Organization
PAHO   Pan American Health Organization
PPP   Purchasing Power Parity
WFME   World Federation for Medical Education
WHO   World Health Organization
UNDP   United Nations Development Programme
UNICEF United Nations Children's Fund
USAID   United States Agency for International Development

FOREWORD

The health workforce crisis is increasingly prominent on the agendas of both developing and developed countries and is a central constraint to strengthening national health systems in affected countries. Addressing this crisis poses a formidable challenge.

The World Health Report 2006, Working Together for Health, calls for leadership at national level in carrying forward country strategies and prescribes sustained action over the next decade. This national-level initiative needs to lead in the delivery of appropriate policies for human resources for health in national health workforce planning. Such policy development necessitates a diversity of expertise, including adequate workforce management systems and tools.

Multilateral and bilateral agencies, donor countries, nongovernmental organizations and the academic community are exploring a common human resources for health framework and tools to support the effort in addressing the HRH crisis and to best respond to the reality faced by countries.

An important part of WHO's mandate is to support countries by providing such tools and guidelines and by facilitating processes aiming to develop health systems with universal coverage and effective public health interventions. Created in collaboration with the International Health Systems Programme of the Harvard School of Public Health, this tool is part of WHO's efforts to fulfill that mandate in recognition of the need for an updated assessment tool for health workforce development.

The tool provides a guidance for the evaluation of the health workforce situation and may be used as a guide for the development of health workforce strategies. The methodology used builds on existing tools and in addition takes into account the changing context and challenges of the 21st century, distilling a wealth of experience in responding to health workforce policy, strategy and planning. The tool can serve as a baseline assessment and evaluator of policy changes as well as a resource for updating and ensuring better understanding of the health workforce context.

Prior to publication and wider dissemination, the tool was tested in a few countries. The authors received contributions and comments at various stages and thanks are extended to James Buchan, Gilles Dussault, Norbert Dreesch, Peter Hornby, Mary O'Neil and Uta Lehman for their revision and comments.

Dr Mario R. Dal Poz

Coordinator
Department of Human Resources for Health
Cluster of Health Systems and Services
World Health Organization

INTRODUCTION

The importance of effective human resources policies for improving the performance of health systems has been increasingly highlighted in recent years (Martinez & Martineau, 1998; Joint Learning Initiative, 2004, WHR 2006). However, health workforce strategic planning and policy development faces two challenges. First, human resources planning has not historically been a policy priority of health ministries in developing countries. It is likely to take slow pace and a much more compelling evidence base to convince health ministries to change their priorities. Second, where such planning has taken place, it has generally focused on inputs and outputs or the staffing needs of specific health programmes. Thus pre-service education and ratios of health workers to target population are often emphasized above all else. While education and deployment figures are important, they are only two components of a much larger set of issues affecting health workforce policies. Broader concerns include financing and payment, the overall educational environment, the management of the health workforce, working conditions, and the policy environment. A more comprehensive approach to designing health workforce policies is therefore warranted.

This document contains a method for assessing the financial, educational and management systems and policy context, essential for strategic planning and policy development for human resources for health. This tool has been developed as an evidence-based comprehensive diagnostic aid to inform policy-making in low and middle income countries in regard to human resources for health. It does so in three stages, by:
- assessing the current status of the health workforce and capacities for health workforce policy implementation with a particular focus on four aspects — finance, education, management, and policy-making;
- identifying priority requirements and actions based on the current status of the health workforce;
- showing how to sequence policies and draw up a prioritized action plan for human resources for health.

This tool is not intended to assess the appropriateness of a workforce's skills mix or the technical quality of pre-service curricula, which are the subjects of several other assessment tools.[1] Rather, it focuses on determining – and providing sequenced recommendations to improve upon – system capacities to increase the effectiveness of the health workforce.

The tool is designed as an initial diagnostic instrument to be used in a process of developing a national strategic plan on human resources for health. It helps to provide a rapid initial assessment and a preliminary strategic plan as part of a longer-term and sustained process of human resources planning.

CONTENT OF THE TOOL

This tool presents an overall framework for assessing system determinants of effective human resources in health, which in turn must be judged by broader objectives of the health system. The ultimate objective of any health intervention is to improve the health status of the population. Recently, however, it has become clear that health interventions should also focus on reducing the financial risk of ill-health, especially for poor people, and should be responsive to stakeholders, patients and the general public (WHO, 2000). In order to achieve these ultimate objectives, it is recognized that intermediate "system goals" of improved equity, quality, efficiency, accessibility, and sustainability need to be addressed.[2] The framework presented here focuses on how the health system components related to the health workforce contribute to these ultimate and intermediate objectives.

We identify a simple, idealized causal chain that, working backwards from the intermediate objectives, specifies the *state of human resources* – the number and type of human resources, their distribution and performance as an output of *cross-cutting issues* such as migration, the attractiveness of professions, and worker motivation, which

---

[1] While the appropriateness and technical quality of curricula for physicians, nurses, front-line workers and other health personnel are important, this tool relies on other studies and experts to attend to those issues. See, for example, Hornby & Forte (2000).

[2] This framework draws upon the work of Roberts (2004) for assessing health system performance in relation to the health workforce. It is consistent with the WHO framework described in WHO (2000).

in turn can be the result of the *policy levers* of changes in financing, education, management systems, and the process of policy change itself (see Figure 1).

The tool provides indicators of the current state of human resources, cross-cutting issues and the policy levers of financing, education and management. These indicators are a means of *identifying problems* that can be addressed by the strategic planning of human resources, and to *provide a baseline* to assess progress towards improving the health system.

The tool is based on a review of the best current evidence for the relationship between changes in the indicators for the various policy levers and their effect on the elements of the causal chain described above. It should be recognized that this *evidence-based approach* is limited by the relatively small number of well-designed studies of these causal links. The current available evidence is presented in annexes and encourage the use of this evidence in arguments to support the policy recommendations that should come out of the analysis outlined in Part 3.

Figure 1 presents a graphic flow chart of this idealized causal chain and an example to illustrate its use in a specific case. As an example, low educational capacity to train a highly skilled health workforce may reduce the attractiveness of the health-related professions compared to jobs in other sectors. These factors can result in a dearth of health workers available for deployment in the health system. An insufficient level of health workers may then compromise service quality or coverage of health services, eventually negatively affecting population health status.

Not all cross-cutting problems (e.g. premature death) are specifically linked to financial, educational, management or policy factors. In other cases, more than one such factor may influence a particular cross-cutting problem (e.g. migration could be affected equally by all four factors). The framework (Figure 1) therefore seeks to provide an understanding of how each of the policy levers may be affecting a variety of factors important for health systems performance.

Figure 1. Strategic planning tool: conceptual framework for assessing human resources for health (HRH)

Policy levers →	Cross-cutting problems →	State of HRH →	System goals →	Health goals
Financing Education Management Policy-making	Profession attractiveness Migration HIV/AIDS epidemic Multiple job holding Absenteeism and ghost workers Motivation	**HRH density level** (how many?) • HRH category **HRH distribution** (where? who?) • Within-category skill-mix • Geographical location • Sector • Gender **HRH performance** (what do they do? how do they do it?) • Quality (clinical; service) • Efficiency	Quality Efficiency Equity/ accessibility Sustainability	Health status Fair financing Responsiveness
Example: Education				
Low number of middle school/ high school graduates, leading to	Limited health professions applicant pool, leading to	Insufficient HRH level, leading to	Compromised quality/equity, leading to	Unsatisfactory population health status

TIMELINE FOR APPLYING THE TOOL

The tool requires some lead time for collecting data and preparing the team for an exercise in analysis of data and strategic planning. It is likely that several months will be needed to sensitize the national team and train them in the basic methods and data collection techniques. If the resources and time of officials are limited, it may be necessary to involve a team of international consultants to do the initial training and to assist in the analysis, and the preparation of reports and seminars for dissemination of information. While the tool is designed to minimize the need for international support, it is important to ensure that the capacity exists to carry out a complete and detailed review of key indicators, given the types of data available and the short period devoted to this initial assessment. We envisage that implementation of this tool will be followed by more detailed assessments of requirements and capabilities as part of longer-term and sustained strategic planning for human resources.

Figure 2 presents the organization and timeline of the tool. During Phase I, a desktop review is undertaken to collect data on the state of a country's health workforce, as well as contextual factors which may eventually constrain human resources policies in the health sector (e.g. disease profile, macroeconomic conditions). During Phases I and II, the desktop review and in-country consultations at the national level will permit implementation of the assessments of human resources for health in terms of the various policy levers. Choice of data to be collected in regard to the policy levers will depend in part on the context and on the data already collected for the needs assessment. During Phases II and III, in-country consultations at both the national and sub-national levels will permit more extensive data collection and probing of priority areas. Phase III will also include identification of priority actions and proposed sequencing of actions.

Figure 2. Timeline for assessing human resources for health (HRH)

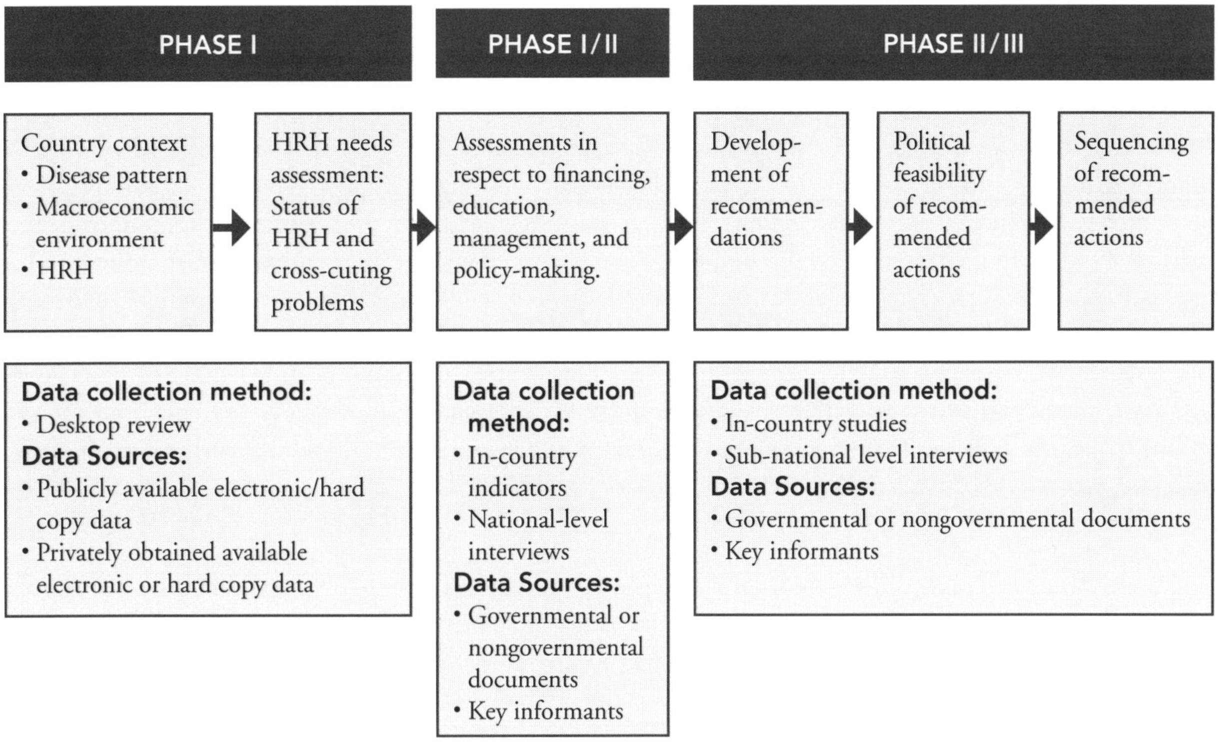

ANALYSES

The following sections describe each component of the three phases in greater detail. In each of the components, *menus of diagnostic indicators* are proposed to assess the various elements related to the health workforce. These indicators have been selected on the basis of three criteria: theoretical or empirical relationships to human resources for health; adaptability of indicators from previous human resources instruments; and practical realities of data collection. Obviously, the appropriateness or feasibility of collecting data on certain indicators will vary by country. Recognizing this reality, the main text includes *primary indicators*, which are the most widely relevant, the most likely to be available, or for which approximate estimates are most likely to be able to be made. The annexes contain other indicators (*secondary indicators*) to supplement the primary or core indicators. The primary indicators are necessary for developing a meaningful strategic plan. If data for these primary indicators are not available, estimates should be made on the basis of judgments by national and international experts. The secondary indicators are to be used when available in order to make a more refined assessment – particularly for quality and management issues. Ultimately, the goal should be to triangulate information in a way appropriate to a country's particular context. Whenever necessary, and insofar as it is feasible, alternative indicators can be substituted for the indicators suggested in this tool, in order to provide the best assessment of the situation of human resources for health in the country concerned.

Status of the health workforce

Part 1 covers the overall assessment of health workforce requirements. This serves as a starting point for assessment (covered in Part 2) of the policy levers: financing, education, management and policy-making. The overall requirements assessment looks first at the status of human resources for health – i.e. the health workforce *level* (adequate number of human resources), *distribution*, and *performance* – as well as cross-cutting problems that may influence the status of human resources for health.

Health workforce requirements are defined as the *gap between the current status* of human resources for health (or the projected status given continuation of current conditions) and the *desired state* of human resources for health in each category of health worker. The assessment of health workforce requirements at this stage does not take into account resource constraints (such as capacity for training or financing human resources for health). Rather, a comparison of the actual status of the health workforce as compared to an ideal or, at least, a benchmarked standard, enables the development of a *prioritized action plan* for human resources for health. It is the final action plan which takes into account both the results of the assessments and the resource constraints facing a given country.

By assessing health workforce requirements, a set of *quantitative targets* are generated which subsequently help to focus and inform the implementation of the policy levers. An overall shortage of nurses, for example, may focus the assessment of policy levers on a particular concern, such as the number of candidates trained or the political response to migration. A surplus of nurses coupled with poor distribution, however, could result in a different emphasis, such as upgrading management capacities to staff facilities with an appropriate skills mix. The target-driven assessment of requirements therefore provides an objective means to evaluate a country's current situation regarding human resources for health. It is both comparable with benchmarks from other country contexts and over time within the same country. As with all stages of data collection in this tool, it will be important early in the process to assess the *quality and reliability of existing data* on the current status of human resources for health and on epidemiological profiles. Evidence of poor quality of data should be acknowledged and forms of estimation explained.

This tool assumes that other existing tools have established targets for the number and type of health professionals and paraprofessionals that are needed to achieve health status and patient satisfaction goals. Information needed for these requirements assessments will vary according to the projection method used. Ideally, the assessment of health workforce requirements should be based on a country's health care needs, taking into account the country's epidemiological profile and projections of its future development needs, given its current path. Alternatively, the assessment of health workforce requirements may have to rely on proxy measures. Indicators of met and unmet demand for health care – such as length of waiting times for certain services, or use rates in different regions of the country – are examples of such measures. Additionally, current and projected health care needs or demand will have to be translated into current and future ideal densities of health workers, by category. Such an analysis may be data intensive, requiring information not only on current densities of health workers, but also on current and projected attrition or entry rates, measures of productivity, and average weekly hours worked, by category.

The planning method used for estimating human resources requirements typically involve *two basic components*: (a) determining the *appropriate number and types* of health services to be offered; and (b) determining the *timeframe* in which health interventions need to be delivered. The most common methods have included: a needs-based approach in which the health workforce or service requirements are estimated on the basis of trends in mortality, morbidity and health gaps; demand-based assessments which incorporate expected demographic trends into current service use; fixing desired health worker-to-population ratios; and setting targets for service delivery, then converting those targets into health workforce requirements. More recently, methods have emerged which combine elements of the four approaches, such as an approach using needs, service targets, time and productivity as a basis for estimates of health workforce requirements, and an adjusted service target approach which incorporates such data inputs as training programme needs and required skills for various tasks related to the Millennium Development Goals.

While determining the requirements for the health workforce is a basic building block of any country's policy on human resources for health, such an exercise is beyond the scope of this tool. For a further analysis of workforce planning methods and approaches related to human resources for health, and for a comprehensive overview and references to appropriate instruments, see Joint Learning Initiative (2004) and Dreesch et al. (2005).

If time and resources or information availability do not allow a fully-fledged assessment of health workforce requirements, a comparison of current health worker densities with external standards (for instance, for the geographical region) may provide a first pass assessment of requirements for human resources. Examples of external standards include:

- health workforce densities (e.g. one physician per 5000 population)
- worker-to-worker ratios (e.g. two nurses per physician)
- worker-to-resource ratios (e.g. one full-time nurse per ten beds)
- worker-to-programme ratios (e.g. two community health workers per health centre programme) (Hall, 2001).

These measures, however, are less than ideal because they are based on the assumption that the denominator measure (population, other professionals, facilities) already reflects health care requirements. In many countries, health care needs are complex, and the distribution of health facilities and human resources may not address the existing health problems.

Policy levers potentially affecting human resources for health

A country's health workforce situation may be improved in a number of ways, from producing more human resources trained with specific skill sets to implementing performance-based management practices. Part 2 focuses on four major policy levers for human resources for health: financing, education, management and policy-making. Based on the available evidence, each of these policy levers is hypothesized to affect the health workforce situation – and therefore health sector performance – in many different ways.

Part 2 of this tool describes pathways between each of the policy levers and the levels, distribution and performance of the health workforce, as well as cross-cutting problems affecting what we call the *status of human resources for health*. A few comments about methods can usefully be made here. For each of the policy levers, we provide an extensive basket of quantitative indicators which have been used in previous studies or assessments, are otherwise documented in the literature, or which have been developed for this tool on theoretical grounds. The evidence that justifies the use of these indicators is presented in the annexes. Wherever possible, benchmarks accompany quantitative indicators. As will be noted throughout, there are many indicators for which there is no literature or experience that provides a reasonable benchmark. It would be useful to begin to develop data and studies to provide benchmarks for these indicators, especially the core indicators. Because it is not expected that every indicator will be applicable or available in all contexts, knowledge of a country's circumstances is needed to select the most appropriate indicators and benchmarks among those offered. Some of the needed knowledge will be available from key informant interviews with experienced local officials concerned with human resources for health, and with experts in health financing, management and education. Other knowledge may require rapid surveys, focus groups, or interactions between international and national experts. It is expected that data availability and quality will, to a large degree, drive the final choice of indicators.

While quantitative indicators facilitate eventual target setting, qualitative assessments of the health workforce situation are needed to complement and provide a context for findings. For instance, extreme levels of staff rotation among district managers may adversely affect health systems performance. Without a qualitative assessment of how very high (or very low) levels of rotation are perceived by staff, it would be difficult to know whether rates of staff rotation indicate underlying management problems of turnover (or entrenchment). Qualitative assessments are therefore as integral a part of this tool as the quantitative indicators.

For either class of indicators – quantitative or qualitative – there is a need to caution against drawing conclusions without carefully assessing the situation from as many angles of explanation as possible. For example, the percentage of the health budget allocated to human resources can be a good indicator of the appropriateness of spending on the health workforce relative to other health sector costs.[3] Yet without knowledge of the *absolute* level of spending for the health budget – and, by extension, for spending on human resources for health – it is not possible to know whether the current health sector spending is adequate to improve capacities by implementing recommended actions. Similarly, while a low rate of appropriately qualified applicants to health education institutions may indicate a lack of high school educational capacity, it may also indicate limited training places in nursing or medical schools, or reflect the lack of attractiveness to prospective students of a career in one of the health care professions. In terms of management, stockouts of essential medicines can provide insights into the functioning of the system and the working conditions of health workers. Yet many other less quantifiable aspects also determine such functioning or working conditions (e.g. quality of communication between levels of the system), making reliance on one indicator of logistics management a limited proxy measure. And the highly contextual nature of a political assessment requires the researcher to use locally relevant sources of information to determine players' positions and power.

This tool is thus designed to "triangulate" information and provide the assessment team with a comprehensive approach to strategic planning and policy-making for improving human resources for health, and hence health system capacities. The range of indicators provided should therefore be used with such an approach in mind, and should be adapted to country-specific concerns where this would be helpful in understanding health workforce outcomes, the status of human resources for health, and the factors influencing health workers.

Policy development for human resources for health

Part 3 of this tool identifies the strategies/solutions and sequencing developed from examining the four policy levers for human resources for health: financing, education, management and policy-making. Part 3 presents general guidelines for reviewing the current status against benchmarks, prioritizing the problem areas, selecting technically and politically feasible policies, and developing a sequencing guide for implementing the policies. We recommend that the material and evidence presented in Parts 1 and 2, as well as in the annexes, form the basis for the activities outlined in Part 3.

The annexes are designed to provide more detailed evidence for the indicators that are described in the body of the text. We provide this evidence so that health workforce analysts will be able to present more detailed evidence for their assessments and more convincing explanations for why the indicators are important when the results of this assessment are presented to policy-makers.

The annexes also present additional (secondary) indicators and their benchmarks. The secondary indicators tend to come from studies in high income countries, and are less likely to be available in low and middle income countries. They would be useful, if available, in providing a more sophisticated analysis of each of the policy levers.

---

[3] It is important to include the budget for training of health professionals, which is often not covered in the ministry of health budget but must be gleaned from the ministry of education and other government budgets. If possible, some estimate of private sector or nongovernmental organizational expenditure on human resources for health should also be made. National Health Accounts may provide rough guides for these estimates.

PART 1 | Status of human resources for health

Explicit and well-designed policies for human resources for health constitute an important mechanism by which governments may improve health system performance. Policies may affect the current state of human resources for health along three broad dimensions:

- density level (the number of health workers in different professional, administrative and support categories);
- distribution and composition (intra-*national* distribution of human resources across geographical regions, skill categories and personal or institutional characteristics, and intra-*organizational* distribution of skill sets or cadres);
- performance (what the health workers do and how they do it).

The following section reviews these dimensions. It presents the categories, and indicators, and briefly explains the policy implications of the potential findings of different levels, distribution and performance in the countries applying this assessment methodology. The tables present the assessment indicators, existing benchmarks, references for evidence for the indicators, and comments on the indicators and potential sources for those indicators to assist the assessment teams in their data collection.

LEVEL OF HUMAN RESOURCES FOR HEALTH

The first task of assessment teams is to determine the numbers of health workers in specific job categories relative to populations being served. These *density levels* are a starting point for all assessments of human resources in any country. Normally these data exist, although they are often estimates, since registration of active practitioners is often not up to date or complete.

Benchmarking what should be an "adequate" density level however is seldom easy. Recently, there have been attempts to posit international minimum standards for some health cadres. For instance, World Health Report 2006 suggests a minimum of 2.3 health workers per 1,000 people is required to "attain adequate coverage of some essential health interventions and core MDG-related health services" (WHO, 2006). Although the empirical links between health-worker levels and health systems performance are not always well-documented, it seems clear that in many developing countries professional staffing levels are inadequate for the populations being served (see Annex 1 for further discussion on the evidence base).

Beyond the proposed standards for physicians and in some cases nurses, there is little guidance in the international literature on "other health workers" – dentists, pharmacists, etc. – and on administrative and other support staff. Ideally, we should disaggregate these categories into the myriad professionals and paraprofessionals, including community-level health workers, administrators and other support staff. In some countries there may be enough information to develop this detailed assessment, but there is not sufficient comparative information to identify key benchmark indicators and the relationships among them for the purposes of the current assessment tool.

The following table presents three indicators, with the current benchmarks for two of them that should form the basis for assessing the density level of different health cadres. The assessment teams might disaggregate the "other" category into specific job categories (including administrative staff) if the country data allow that to be done, but there are no general benchmarks for these categories.

Table 1. Status of human resources for health (HRH): primary indicators of HRH density level

Dimension	Indicator	Bench-mark	Reference	Comments	
				Indicator/benchmark(s)	Source
• HRH level	Number of physicians/per 10 000 population	None	*Benchmark:* • No international benchmarks	1.0: minimum package of clinical and public health interventions 2.0: "Health For All" value	Can be assessed through internationally-accessible databases, in-country databases or ministry of health documents
• HRH level	Number of nurses per 10000 population	None	*Benchmark:* • No international benchmarks		Can be assessed through internationally-accessible databases, in-country databases or ministry of health documents
• HRH level	Number of other HRH categories (e.g. dentists) per 10 000 population	None	*Benchmark:* • No international benchmarks	Other categories include, but are not limited to: midwives, health assistants, front-line workers, physician specialists, pharmacists, administrators, other support staff	Can be assessed through internationally-accessible databases, in-country databases or ministry of health documents

DISTRIBUTION OF HUMAN RESOURCES FOR HEALTH

The average density levels may mask significant differences in the distribution of human resources along geographic, skills, gender and sectoral dimensions. These distributional differences may be some of the most important obstacles to achieving the broad goals of improved health status in a population, citizen satisfaction and sustainable financial protection. Geographical imbalances usually imply a clustering of the health workforce in cities, and therefore scarcity of health workers in rural areas. In general, international literature posits an objective of more equity for geographic distribution, although few countries are able to achieve this benchmark. There are a range of policy options for addressing this imbalance through incentives and regulations, which have been only marginally effective.

Skills imbalances, for instance the ratios of nurses to doctors, or unskilled to skilled human resources, may also reflect differences in availability and quality of services. However, comparative analyses of these ratios show no consistent pattern among countries and no clear justification of benchmarks for the different ratios. It is likely that a more detailed assessment of the tasks and skills for different categories along with an economic analysis of the cost-effectiveness of different skill mixes is necessary to develop country benchmarks.

Gender distribution, which results in clustering of women and men in certain health professions, such as physicians being predominantly male and nurses and lower-status staff being predominantly female, may have some justification for certain categories where female patients are more comfortable with female providers. In general, however, recent literature promotes more equity in this indicator.

Sector differences may be assessed by determining the ratio of private to public sector health workers. While there are no guidelines for this ratio, it may be important in determining the policy options for access for poor people, regulating quality of services, and determining subsidy policies.

Distributional imbalances are felt to entail a number of adverse consequences, including: the brain drain from public rural to private urban centres; inattention to gender-specific health problems and patterns of service use; lower quality and productivity of health services; increased waiting time and reduced numbers of available hospital beds; and certain interventions being carried out by lower-qualified personnel (Zurn et al., 2002; Gupta et al., 2003; Wibulpolprasert & Pengpaibon, 2003).

The following table presents the indicators, benchmarks, references, and potential sources of data for the assessment of distribution of health workers.

Table 2. Status of human resources for health (HRH): primary indicators of HRH distribution

Dimension	Indicator	Bench-mark	Reference	Comments	
				Indicator/ benchmark(s)	Source
• HRH geographic distribution	Ratio highest: lowest physician densities by region	1.0	*Benchmark:* • 1.0: equity rationale		Can be assessed through internationally-accessible databases, in-country databases or ministry of health documents
• HRH geographic distribution	Ratio highest: lowest nurse densities by region	1.0	*Benchmark:* • 1.0: equity rationale		Can be assessed through internationally-accessible databases, in-country databases or ministry of health documents
• HRH geographic distribution	Ratio highest: lowest other HRH densities by region	1.0	*Benchmark:* • 1.0: equity rationale	Other categories include, but are not limited to: midwives, health assistants, front-line workers, physician specialists, pharmacists, administrators and other support staff	Can be assessed through internationally-accessible databases, in-country databases or ministry of health documents
• HRH gender distribution	Ratio male: female by HRH category	None		Categories include, but are not limited to: physicians, nurses, midwives, health assistants, front-line workers, physician specialists, pharmacists, administrators and other support staff	Can be assessed through internationally-accessible databases, in-country databases or ministry of health documents
• HRH skills distribution	Ratio nurses: physicians	2.0	*Benchmark:* • 2.0: World Bank (1994a)		Can be assessed through internationally-accessible databases, in-country databases or ministry of health documents
• HRH skills distribution	Ratio unskilled: skilled HRH	None			Can be assessed through internationally-accessible databases, in-country databases or ministry of health documents
• HRH skills distribution	Ratio public: private providers by HRH category	None		Categories include, but are not limited to: physicians, nurses, midwives, health assistants, front-line workers, physician specialists, pharmacists, administrators and other support staff	Can be assessed through internationally-accessible databases, in-country databases or ministry of health documents

PERFORMANCE OF HUMAN RESOURCES FOR HEALTH

Performance of human resources for health comprises both personnel *efficiency* and provider *quality*. The efficiency of the health workforce may be analysed as *financial efficiency* (e.g. the number of health workers employed per dollar expended) and *productivity* (e.g. the number of services provided per person–hour). Both are important for health systems performance, in terms of making optimum use of scarce resources and containing costs of health workers. The simple gross indicators, however, may mask the impact of other inputs (supplies, facilities) as well as the relationship between quantity and quality of production.

Quality in health care can be divided into two subcategories: *clinical quality* (measured objectively as clinical performance); and *patient satisfaction* (quality measured subjectively as perceived by patients). Clinical quality is crucial in improving health outcomes, while patient satisfaction is an important health system objective in and of itself and may ultimately affect population health as well. While systematic assessments of quality of services are often lacking in many countries, here we identify some basic indicators to indicate general quality levels for different levels of care. Vaccination coverage and certain rates of service use (e.g. use of primary health care) may indicate general quality of care. Stockout rates can be used in general assessments of logistics system quality, and internal infection rates are often an indication of general quality of hospital care.

The following table summarizes several sample indicators and benchmarks as well as the sources for the assessment of the performance of the health workforce.

Table 3. Status of human resources for health (HRH): primary indicators of HRH performance

Dimension	Indicator	Bench-mark	Reference	Comments	
				Indicator/benchmark	Source
• HRH performance (efficiency)	Annual budget for HRH/total annual health budget	None	*Indicator* • Hornby & Forte (2000)		Can be assessed through internationally-accessible databases, in-country databases or ministry of health documents
• HRH performance (efficiency)	Number of HRH by cat-egory/annual budget for HRH in that category	None	*Indicator* • No specific source		Can be assessed through internationally-accessible databases, in-country databases or ministry of health documents
• HRH performance (efficiency)	Total per capita HRH spending	None	*Indicator* • No specific source		Can be assessed through internationally-accessible databases, in-country databases or ministry of health documents
• HRH performance (efficiency)	Average annual earnings by HRH category	None	*Indicator* • Hornby & Forte (2000)		Can be assessed through internationally-accessible databases, in-country databases or ministry of health documents
• HRH performance (productivity)	Average hos-pital length of stay	None	*Indicator* • No specific source		Can be assessed through internationally-accessible databases, in-country databases or ministry of health documents

Dimension	Indicator	Bench-mark	Reference	Comments	
				Indicator/ benchmark	Source
• HRH performance (productiv-ity/quality)	Average number of immunizations administered per day by number of health staff	None	*Indicator* • Hall (2001)	Measure of ability to meet staff productivity targets	Can be assessed through internationally-accessible databases, in-country databases or ministry of health documents
• HRH performance (productiv-ity/quality)	Primary health care attendances / total staff	None	*Indicator* • Hornby & Forte (2000)	Measure of ability to meet staff productivity targets	Can be assessed through internationally-accessible databases, in-country databases or ministry of health documents
• HRH performance (quality)	Stockouts of essential medicines	0%	*Indicator:* • DELIVER/ John Snow (2002) (adapted) *Benchmark:* • 0%: ideal	Indicator of system-level logistics quality (cross-referenced in management section)	Can be assessed through document review (e.g. pharmaceutical management study) or key informant interviews
• HRH performance (quality)	Number of cross-infections / number of hospital patients	0	*Indicator* • Hornby & Forte (2000) *Benchmark:* • 0: ideal		Can be assessed through internationally-accessible databases, in-country databases or ministry of health documents

CROSS-CUTTING PROBLEMS CONCERNING HUMAN RESOURCES FOR HEALTH

In addition to the basic indicators of the state of health workers – their density levels, distribution and general performance – we have identified a series of cross-cutting problems which in turn influence the density, distribution and performance of the workforce. These are problems that are not inherent in the financing, education or management systems but rather are to be addressed by policy changes in these systems. They can be seen as *intermediate* causes of changes and status of the density levels, distribution and performance of the workforce that will be affected by changes in the policy levers of financing, education and management in our scheme presented in Figure 1.

The cross-cutting problems have been identified in much of the literature on the current human resources "crisis" (Joint Learning Initiative, 2004; WHO, 2006). They include the attractiveness of health professions for graduates of pre-professional schools, migration of health professionals to wealthier countries, the threat to the health of health workers posed by the HIV/AIDs epidemic, multiple job holding, absenteeism and low motivation. The core diagnostic indicators for these problems are grouped together in a table at the end of this section.

Attractiveness of health professions for graduates of pre-professional schools

The demand for professional education in the health field is important for determining the density level, distribution and ultimately the performance of the health workforce. Without entrants into medical, nursing and other professional schools, there will not be a sufficient inflow to improve these indicators of the state of the health workforce. It is also important to recognize that the health professions are competing with other professions for highly skilled and motivated graduates and therefore that the quality of the health workforce will be affected by the results of this competition. A student's choice of professional education can be seen as an investment decision in which costs of education are weighed against expected financial returns. In addition to anticipated financial payoffs from choosing to enter the field of health, non-monetary factors may play a part in prospective students' decisions. These latter factors may include perceived working conditions, job security and career development, status of the profession, and intrinsically motivated concerns such as the desire to promote health. Empirical evidence suggests that both monetary and non-monetary benefits do affect entry decisions (see Annex 1 for further discussion on the evidence base).

Migration

Emigration of health personnel to other countries is felt to pose a significant problem to health systems of low and middle income countries. While the free flow of physicians, nurses and other health personnel can increase information sharing and knowledge-building, low income countries are especially vulnerable to a brain drain of their most highly skilled workers. The departure of highly skilled health workers can adversely affect the quality of care in the originating country's health system, and the depletion of human resources could jeopardize future macroeconomic prospects. Although the nature of migration (e.g. temporary versus permanent) plays a large role in its eventual impact, emigration often entails more negative than positive consequences for countries already experiencing shortages in key health personnel (Forcier et al., 2004). Empirical evidence indicates that migration flows are considerable, and emigration from developing countries can entail negative consequences for the level of the health workforce and the efficiency of the health system (see Annex 1 for further discussion on the evidence base).

Health threat to health workers of the HIV/AIDS epidemic

Elevated mortality rates among health professionals, in particular from the HIV/AIDS epidemic, can be a significant drain on human capital and financial resources because of the need to replace deceased workers. While the evidence base on this point is limited (see Annex 1), lessons may be drawn from other social sectors. In the education sector, for instance, the required replacement of professionals who die from HIV/AIDS outstrips countries' capacities (Cohen, 2002). Similarly, health systems, particularly in Africa, face morbidity and the loss of a vast number of trained health workers (Tawfik, 2006). In addition, the potential threat to the personal health of health workers who treat infected patients (through lack of protection from needle sticks, etc.) may influence choices to enter or remain in the profession and to emigrate to countries with lower incidence of the disease.

Multiple job holding

Multiple job holding in the health sector – simultaneous provision of services by government employees outside their public sector appointment – can lead to a number of problems in the efficiency and quality of care. On the one hand, multiple job holding may decrease productivity in the lower-paying (often public sector) post or even overtax the provider and jeopardize productivity and quality in both jobs. On the other hand, multiple job holding may lead to inappropriate use of public resources for private gain or unnecessary referrals from public to private practice (Ferrinho & Lerberghe, 2000; Ensor & Duran-Moreno, 2002; Berman & Cuizon, 2004). While relationships between multiple job holding and system performance are still not well-understood (see Annex 1 for further discussion on the evidence base), the prevalence of multiple job holding is significant enough to warrant attention in this tool.

Absenteeism and "ghost workers"

Public sector absenteeism and "ghost workers" (personnel posts which exist on paper but not in practice, leading to inappropriate collection of salaries by "ghost" personnel) can adversely affect health system performance by reducing efficiencies (i.e. productivity of health workers per dollar spent and governmental capacity to increase the overall salary level), access (i.e. hours per week that providers treat patients), and quality – clinical and perceived – of care (Chaudhury & Hammer, 2003; Huddart & Picazo, 2003). Absenteeism and ghost workers are known to be significant problems in many contexts, but more research is needed to link these phenomena to health systems performance (see Annex 1 for further discussion on the evidence base).

Motivation

Given that the health sector is human resource intensive by nature, the motivation of health workers plays a key role, alongside their ability, in determining system performance. Health worker motivation may be defined as employee willingness to "exert and maintain an effort towards organizational goals" (Franco et al., 2002) by influencing "workers' allocation of personal resources towards those goals". Motivation in turn affects effectiveness and productivity. Job satisfaction may be a major pathway linking motivation to organizational performance. The inherent difficulties in researching motivation have thus far limited the evidence base linking motivation to system performance (see Annex 1 for further discussion on the evidence base).

Table 4. Cross-cutting problems concerning human resources for health (HRH): primary indicators

Dimension	Indicator	Bench-mark	Reference	Comments	
				Indicator/ benchmark	Source
• Attractive-ness of profession	Number of applicants per HRH category school place	None	None	Categories include, but are not limited to: physicians, nurses, midwives, health assistants, front-line workers, physician specialists, pharmacists, administrators and other support staff	Can be assessed through internationally-accessible databases, in-country databases or ministry of health documents
• Attractive-ness of profession	Estimate of quality of applicants	None	None	Categories include, but are not limited to: physicians, nurses, midwives, health assistants, front-line workers, physician specialists, pharmacists, administrators and other support staff	Can be assessed through internationally-accessible databases, in-country databases, ministry of health documents or by panel of experts or other methods of estimation
• Migration	Annual net in-migration in % by HRH category	None	None	Categories include, but are not limited to: physicians, nurses, midwives, health assistants, front-line workers, physician specialists, pharmacists, administrators and other support staff	Can be assessed through internationally-accessible databases, labour market surveys or other special studies; in-country databases, ministry of health documents, or by panel of experts or other methods of estimation

Dimension	Indicator	Bench-mark	Reference	Comments	
				Indicator/ benchmark	Source
• Migration	Annual net out-migration in % by HRH category	None	None	Categories include, but are not limited to: physicians, nurses, midwives, health assistants, front line workers, physician specialists, pharmacists, administrators and other support staff	Can be assessed through internationally-accessible databases, labour market surveys or other special studies, in-country databases, ministry of health documents, or by panel of experts or other methods of estimation
• Premature death	Average rate of HIV/AIDS deaths by HRH category	None	None	Categories include, but are not limited to: physicians, nurses, midwives, health assistants, front line workers, physician specialists, pharmacists, administrators and other support staff	Can be assessed through internationally-accessible databases, in-country databases, ministry of health documents or by panel of experts or other methods of estimation
• Multiple job holding	Proportion of physicians working in more than one health care job	None	None		Can be assessed through internationally-accessible databases, in-country databases, ministry of health documents, or by panel of experts or other methods of estimation
• Multiple job holding	Proportion of other HRH categories working in more than one health care job	None	None	Other categories include, but are not limited to: nurses, midwives, health assistants, front line workers, physician specialists, pharmacists, administrators and other support staff.	Can be assessed through internationally-accessible databases, in-country databases, ministry of health documents, or by panel of experts or other methods of estimation
• Absentee-ism and "ghost workers"	HRH absence rate (aggregate)	None	None		Can be assessed through in-country studies, in-country databases, ministry of health documents, or by panel of experts or other methods of estimation
• Absentee-ism and "ghost workers"	Average number of hours worked per week per HRH category	None	None		Can be assessed through previous in-country studies, in-country databases, ministry of health documents, or by panel of experts or other methods of estimation
• Motivation	Qualitative indicator: views on the extent to which motivation is a problem	None	None		Can be assessed through previous in-country studies, key informant interviews or other methods of estimation

PART 2 Policy levers affecting human resources for health

FINANCING

One of the most important factors influencing the cross-cutting problems and the state of the health workforce is the financing available to pay salaries and the other important non-salary inputs needed for the effectiveness of the health system. In this section we introduce indicators to assess the appropriateness of the levels of financing of salaries, the relation of salaries to non-salary inputs, and the envelope of national economic resources available for these expenditures.

The salaries of human resources for health are usually the most important determinant of recurrent health care expenditures.[1] Relative to other health expenditures, such as drugs and other supplies, salaries of these individual providers tend to absorb a major portion of all spending in the health sector. Saltman & Von Otter (1995) estimate that the total salary level in most countries accounts for 65% to 80% of recurrent health care expenditures.[2] This proportion may be particularly high in health care systems with a large proportion of care at the primary and community level, since the cost of drugs and other supplies at this level of care is usually low (Pong et al., 1995).

In turn, the *salary level* – as well as the level of non-salary inputs such as drugs and other supplies, which usually vary directly with levels of health workers – are among the most important determinants of a health care system's performance, influencing the level, distribution and performance of health workers in a country (Diallo et al., 2003). It is also important to recognize that as the portion of recurrent funds devoted to the health workforce increases, the resources available for other critical inputs, such as drugs and supplies, may decline significantly, undermining quality of service and making working conditions more difficult. Higher expenditures on the health workforce will in turn influence the ability of the system to achieve higher levels of the intermediate objectives: health system efficiency and sustainability, and financial protection of health system users. Higher levels of expenditures on health workers will lead to higher total health care expenditure, possibly decreasing the health care system's efficiency and ability to offer financial protection to citizens in the long run. The salary level and the level of non-salary expenditures on the health workforce thus need to be determined by balancing the financial efficiency goal of the health care system as a whole with the need to optimize the level, distribution and performance of health workers.[3]

While financial assessments of human resources for health are often confined to an evaluation of the salary or wage bill, analysts should also be prepared to judge the appropriateness of *selected non-salary expenditures* in achieving health workforce goals. Given the large number of potentially relevant non-salary expenditures on human resources for health, such a selection will enable analysts to identify those important financial levers that may be more effective in achieving health workforce goals than salary changes, while maintaining the rapidity of the analysis. For this purpose, the second section of this module provides a checklist of those non-salary health care expenditures that are likely to affect the level, distribution, or performance of a country's health workforce. Selected individual items of expenditure can be analysed following the same logic as the analysis of the salary levels.

---

[1] We use the term "salary" to include all sources of income to the health workforce (salaries, bonuses, fees, etc.) for which there are data. Some economists use the term "wage bill" for this concept.

[2] For Africa, Huddart & Picazo (2003) estimate that 50% to 70% of recurrent health care expenditures are spent on human resources for health.

[3] More detailed discussion of two specific financing needs for human resources for health can be found in the discussions of the financing of education and training, and of financial incentives as a management tool.

If it is determined that expenditures (salary and non-salary) on the health workforce need to be increased, an assessment also needs to be made as to whether and how such an increase can be financed given the macroeconomic constraints in the country. The third section of this module provides a framework to rapidly assess a country's capacity to finance increases in health workforce expenditures.

Salary levels of health workers

The current salary levels for health workers in a country can be analysed by answering the following questions:
- Are salary levels high enough in order to attain health goals?
- Are salary levels producing appropriate levels of services? Or putting that question in economic terms: are they operationally (or technically) efficient?
- Relative to other expenditures, are salary levels appropriate? Or putting that question in economic terms: are they allocatively efficient?

The first component of this section provides diagnostic indicators to answer the first question with regard to the status, level, distribution and performance of the health workforce in a country. The second component offers a diagnostic framework to answer the second and third questions.

Salary level as a determinant of level, distribution and performance of health workers

Salaries are an important determinant of the level, distribution and performance of health workers. Low salaries may discourage entry into some categories of health work, fail to attract health workers to rural areas, and lead to low motivation to improve efficiency and quality of performance. They also affect several of the cross-cutting problems, especially multiple job holding and migration to countries with much higher salary levels.

To assess the effect of salaries, it is often useful to benchmark salaries in similar professions, to consider the difference between salaries in the private and public sectors, and to take account of health workers' perceptions of the adequacy of the salary level.

Increasing salaries or targeting them in order to provide incentives for improved performance or for service in underserved areas are strategies that often can increase the chances of achieving the objectives of health systems. It is important, however, to design payment mechanisms so that they will improve efficiency at the same time as addressing worker motivation and satisfaction. Salary increases that do not provide incentives and motivation for better service may resolve retention problems at the cost of other objectives (see Annex 2 for further discussion on the evidence base).

There are no clear benchmarks to establish an optimal level of spending on salaries for a country; however, per capita expenditure on salaries is often cited in national human resources figures. To assess whether too much or too little is being spent on salaries for the health workforce in a rapid assessment, the amount spent on the health workforce per capita may be compared to the amount spent in other countries with a similar disease burden and at a similar level of economic development.

Allocative and operational efficiency

In assessing the financing of human resources for health it is important to evaluate whether the funding is being used efficiently. This important question is not easy to answer and involves at least two concepts: (a) whether the salaries are producing the highest levels of services for the funding (operational efficiency); and (b) whether the salaries are the right thing to be funding for achieving health objectives (allocative efficiency).

The decision tree in Figure 3 offers a framework for assessing both the allocative efficiency and the operational efficiency of the health workforce salary levels. While it would be ideal to establish whether a country's health workforce salary levels are efficient using specialized studies of health worker productivity, such studies are seldom available in low and middle income countries. For this tool, broader indicators will probably have to be used to determine the efficiency of spending on salaries.

Figure 3. Allocative and operational efficiency of the salaries for the health workforce

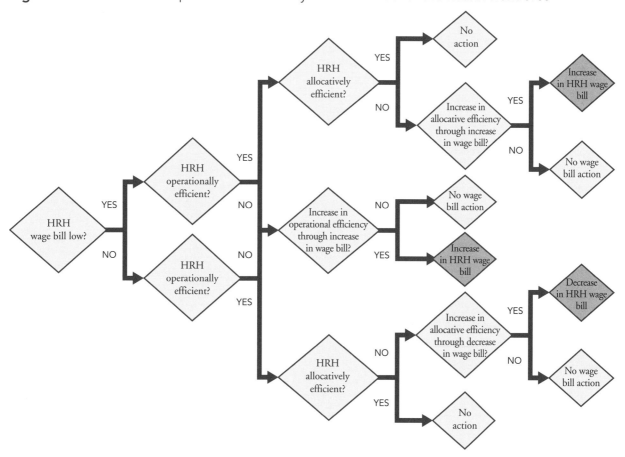

There are two possible sources of operational inefficiency of the health workforce salary levels. First, salary levels may be too high. In other words, the same health outcomes could be achieved if a country's health workers earned less. Whether this is likely to be the case may be found out, for instance, by benchmarking health workers' salaries against salaries earned by health workers in comparable countries or against salaries earned by other professions requiring a similar level of education as health workers in the country of analysis, or more simply by examining the relationship between the average salary of the health workforce and per capita gross domestic product (GDP). Second, if the salary levels are as low as possible to recruit a given number of health workers, the salary level would be operationally inefficient if the health workers do not achieve their maximum productivity with regard to health goals. Whether this is likely to be the case may be judged, for instance, by comparing the level of achievement of intermediate health outcomes in different regions of a country as a function of those regions' density of health workers (ideally controlling for other important factors that could influence health outcomes).[4] For example, if the attainment of public health goals such as childhood vaccination coverage is negatively associated with health worker density across different regions of a country (controlling for regional education, income, average distance to a health care facility, and health care spending other than spending on health workers), it is likely that the health workers in a region with low childhood vaccination coverage work in a way that is operationally inefficient with regard to the health goal of achieving universal childhood vaccination coverage. This could be measured indirectly by assessing the densities of health workers (as a proxy for their salary levels) in relation to the incidence of disease (see Annex 2 for further discussion on the evidence base).

If the salary level for the health workforce is operationally efficient, a high salary level could result from spending which is allocatively inefficient, for instance if too much is spent on the health workforce relative to other health care inputs or if too much is spent on one category of health worker relative to other categories. Examples of

---

[4] If health workers' productivity is a function of the salary level, the optimal salary level may not be the minimum salary level at which a health worker may be recruited.

indicators that may suggest an allocative inefficiency of the health workforce salary levels are the ratio of doctors to nurses or the ratio of community health workers to community health clinics.

Judging whether human resources for health are allocatively efficient involves a variety of factors, such as the balance between different categories (e.g. the balance between specialists, general practitioners and nurses), as discussed above in relation to the performance of the health workforce. In this rapid assessment, broader economic measures of the allocative efficiency of financing will be used. In this section, the level of spending on the health workforce relative to total health expenditure can be taken as a general indicator of allocative efficiency, since higher expenditures on salaries tend to crowd out expenditures on the non-salary inputs needed for health workers to be effective. Other indicators of allocative efficiency are the proportion of GDP dedicated to health and the per capita expenditure on health. These indicators suggest the allocation of general economic resources to health and are the boundaries within which health workforce salary expenditures are assigned.

Using Figure 3, a diagnosis can be made as to whether a country's salary level is likely to be too high or too low as judged by estimates of the allocative and operational efficiency of the expenditure on salaries. Similarly, the appropriateness of any other expenditure item relevant to the health workforce can be assessed (see, for instance, the following section on non-salary expenditures). Moving from left to right along the decision tree, the binary decisions made at each decision node (efficient versus not inefficient) can be guided by different categories of benchmarks:

- *Benchmarking to other countries.* Salary levels in countries which have achieved their objectives with re-gard to the status of human resources for health can serve as a comparison in order to determine optimal salary levels. Cross-country comparison will be the more meaningful the more similar the comparison country is to the country in which the benchmarking exercise takes place, along a number of dimensions, including culture, type of health care system, health care needs, and a number of socioeconomic measures, such as GDP, poverty levels, and education. In addition, benchmarking to other countries has the advantage that it is a comparatively quick method of evaluating health workforce financing levels in a country, because National Health Accounts and other sources for different types of health care expenditures are often readily available. Salary levels need to be adjusted for purchasing power parity in order to allow for meaningful cross-country comparison.
- *Benchmarking to other times.* If a country has time-series data for some of the indicators described above, the salary levels (adjusted for inflation and, possibly, salaries in other professions at the same time) can be used as benchmarks for any of the areas of health-system performance.
- *Benchmarking to other professions.* Salaries in professions which have desired levels of applicant density and quality, net out-migration, job change and job satisfaction, may serve as a benchmark for health workforce salaries. Since performance levels across professions are hard to compare, and opportunities for multiple job holding are very different in different professions, cross-professional comparison in these two areas will be less likely to be meaningful.
- *Benchmarking to political target.* If a country has established a political target with regard to an indicator, the indicator value needs to be benchmarked against that target in order to assure buy-in to recommenda-tions derived from the benchmarking exercise.

The salary decision tree leads to a diagnosis as to whether the health workforce salary level is:
- too high, leading to a decision to decrease the overall salary level;
- too low, leading to a decision to increase salary levels;
- appropriate, leading to a decision that there will be no action on salary levels.

The core diagnostic indicators for use in assessing the financing of human resources for health are given in the following table.

Table 5. Financing of human resources for health (HRH): primary indicators

Dimension	Indicator	Bench-mark	Reference	Comments	
				Indicator/ benchmark	Source
• Salary level	Average salary level of HRH by HRH category	None	None	Benchmark types: • Cross-profession • Cross-country • Comparison to regional cost of living Additional information: • Perception of HRH of their salary level • Perception of HRH of salary levels in other countries or professions	Can be assessed through: internationally-accessible databases; in-country databases or ministry of health documents
• Attractive-ness of HRH professions: salary level	Ratio of HRH salary levels to comparable professionals (e.g. lawyers, teachers)	None	None	Additional information: • Reasons given by recent middle and high school graduates why they did or did not choose an HRH profession as a career	Can be assessed through internationally-accessible databases or in-country databases
• Geographi-cal distri-bution: salary level	Average salary ratio in rural : urban areas, by HRH category	None	None	Benchmark types: • Cross-profession • Cross-country Additional information: • Reasons given for choos-ing or not choosing rural practice, by HRH category	Can be assessed through internationally-accessible databases or in-country databases
• Gender dis-tribution: salary level	Ratio of average male: female HRH salary levels	1	*Benchmark:* • Equity rationale	Benchmark types: • Cross-country • Politically set target	Can be assessed through: internationally-accessible databases; in-country databases
• Allocative efficiency and HRH financing capacity	Salary level as a proportion of total recur-rent govern-ment expen-diture	65%–80% 50%–70% (Africa)	*Benchmark:* • 65%–80% (Saltman & Von Otter, 1995) • 50%–70% (Huddart & Picazo, 2003)		Can be assessed through National Health Accounts or ministry of health documents
• Allocative efficiency and HRH financing capacity	Total health-care expen-ditures as a proportion of GDP	6.6%–13.9% (OECD) 4%–7.8% (Africa)	*Benchmark:* • 6.6%–13.9% (Huber & Orosz, 2003) • 4%-7.8% (Bossert et al., 2004)		Can be assessed through internationally-acces-sible databases, scientific publications, in-country databases or ministry of health documents

Dimension	Indicator	Bench-mark	Reference	Comments	
				Indicator/ benchmark	Source
• Allocative efficiency and HRH financing capacity	Total per capita health care expenditure in $PPP	1500–4880 (OECD) 112 (East and South African average)	Benchmark: • 1500–4880 (Huber & Orosz, 2003) • 112 (Bossert et al., 2004; Nandakumar et al., 2004)		Can be assessed through internationally-accessible databases, scientific publications; in-country databases or ministry of health documents
• Operational efficiency	HRH salary level in comparison to per capita GDP	1.2 (nurse USA) 3–13 (physician USA) 5–24 (range in sub-Saharan Africa)	Benchmark: • 5–24 (World Bank, 2004)		Can be assessed through internationally-accessible databases, in-country databases or and ministry of health documents
• Operational efficiency	Health outcomes relative to HRH density (e.g. malaria death, Infant mortality rate, Maternal mortality rate)	None	None	Compare Anand & Barnighausen (2004)	Can be assessed through in-country databases, ministry of health documents or scientific publications

Non-salary expenditures

Obviously, the salary level is not the only possible determinant of the level, distribution and performance of the health workforce. A number of other factors will affect the attractiveness of the health care professions or the satisfaction of health workers who currently work in a country. These include such expenditures as insurance, benefits, pensions, and in-service or continuing education opportunities. Figure 4 highlights a number of non-salary expenditures relevant to health workers, and Annex 2 provides a more detailed discussion of the evidence base related to this topic.

The framework used to analyse the appropriateness of the current health workforce salary level can be applied to any non-salary expenditure item as well.

Figure 4. Checklist of non-salary health care expenditures relevant to human resources for health

Category	Examples
Recurrent health care inputs	
Supplies	• Pharmaceuticals • Surgical instruments
Workplace safety measures	• Surgical technologies • Post-exposure HIV prophylaxis • High-quality gloves • High-quality needles and scalpels

Education	• Sub-specializations • Continuing education opportunities
Benefits	• Pension benefits • Child care • Health insurance • Accident insurance
Psychosocial support structures	• Psychological counselling for health workers • Peer support groups
Health care capital inputs	
	• Facilities • Laboratory equipment • Imaging technologies • Surgical technologies

Macroeconomic context

Levels of financing for the health workforce are constrained first by the funding available to the health sector and then by the allocation to health workers within the health sector. Assessment of the allocations to the health sector involves first an overall estimate of health spending as a proportion of GDP, which gives an idea of the total spending in both the public and private sectors. Since policy levers tend to focus on health spending by the national government and donors, it is particularly important to assess both the proportion of the national budget that is devoted to health and the proportion of national health expenditure that is funded by donors. For the health workforce, the most important budget is for recurrent costs, although the capital expenditure budget may affect working conditions and educational opportunities. The National Health Accounts are often a good basis for this kind of analysis.

If the assessments of the densities of health workers or the assessments of the levels and efficiency of expenditure on salaries point to an increase in the number of health workers, then two exercises are needed. First, it is necessary to estimate how much the proposed expansion of the workforce will cost, and second, whether the macroeconomic context and the total spending on health would allow this increase in salary expenditure.

There are many ways to project the financing needs for an increase in human resources for health. For instance, a rough formula for such a calculation might be:

> (number of health workers at baseline) × (increase rate) × (1 − attrition rate) ×(average salary + average recurrent non-salary expenditures per health worker),

> where:
> number of health workers at baseline = the number of health workers (by category) in the current year,
> increase rate = 1 + desired proportional increase in the number of health workers (by category) per year,
> attrition rate = the proportional attrition of health workers (by category) per year.

If the above analysis indicates that an increase in expenditure on the health workforce would be expected to significantly increase the adequacy of a country's level, distribution or performance of health workers, the country's capacity to sustain such an increase will need to be considered. Theoretically, an increase in expenditure on human resources for health could be financed via a number of mechanisms, alone or in combination. An analyst should evaluate which of these different mechanisms are the most feasible sources of an increase in expenditure, given common problems attached to their use. Figure 5 offers a checklist for such an analysis.

If the national economy is growing, an increase in spending on the health workforce may be possible without increasing the proportion of the public budget that is currently spent on human resources for health. However, economic growth may not be high enough to satisfy an additional financing need and may not be sustainable. In the absence of economic growth, the share of GDP (or the public budget) that is spent on human resources for health may certainly be increased. But this implies one or more of the following:

- an increase in health workforce financing as a share of GDP
- revenue generation
- a shift in public spending towards health
- a shift in public health spending towards human resources for health.

An increase in health workforce financing as a share of GDP may not be feasible because the government (or the social insurance funds) may not be able to raise taxes (or contribution rates). Revenue generation (for instance, through user fees), on the other hand, may increase inequity in access to health care. Shifts in spending from another sector to the health care sector may encounter resistance from the relevant stakeholders. A shift in spending within the health care sector, for instance from non-salary spending, is only advisable if it does not result in allocative inefficiency. If donors recognize the need for increased spending on human resources for health, donors may function as a source of finance. However, donor funding is unlikely to be a reliable source for recurrent expenditures in the long run, because donors may not be willing to finance the health workforce salaries or may change their objectives over time. In sum, in analysing possible sources for an increase in health workforce spending, the assessment team will likely need to compare the trade-offs between the benefits of such an increase and its negative side-effects across a range of financing options.

If health workforce expenditures are indeed increased, care must be taken to monitor whether the increase does indeed have the intended effect (e.g. an increase in the level of health workers). An increase without the intended (or any other) beneficial effect would constitute a decrease in operational efficiency.

Figure 5. Checklist of macroeconomic considerations relevant to human resources for health (HRH)

Financing options	Potential problems	Indicators
Economic growth	• Economic growth may not be present • If economic growth is present, it may not be sustainable	• GDP growth rate
Increase HRH financing as a share of GDP	• May either imply an increase in the tax base and contributions to insurance schemes, or a decrease in spending in other sectors	• Current health expenditures as a proportion of GDP
Donor funding	• May not be sustainable	• Proportion of 20 largest donors which explicitly name HRH as one of their priorities in their strategic plans • Proportion of 20 largest donors which have an HRH strategy document published in the past two years
Revenue generation	• May increase inequity in health care financing	• Fees or tariffs as proportion of total health expenditure
Shift public spending towards health	• May encounter resistance from other ministries or sectors	• Health budget as proportion of total public expenditure
Shift public health spending towards HRH	• May not be allocatively efficient	• HRH budget as proportion of public health budget

EDUCATION

A country's health education system should produce an appropriately skilled workforce to address its health priorities. The education system helps to determine two key elements of that workforce: the number of graduates with a given skill set (e.g. physicians, nurses, pharmacists, laboratory technicians, paraprofessionals) and the quality of those human resources (e.g. knowledge and skills). In assessing the role of the education system for strategic planning and policy-making it is important to develop indicators of the quantity and quality of graduates educated in the health professions.

Quantity of graduates

An education system's capacity to provide an adequately trained workforce and an appropriate quantity of health workers can be presented as an "education funnel" (Figure 6).

Figure 6. "Education funnel" for human resources for health

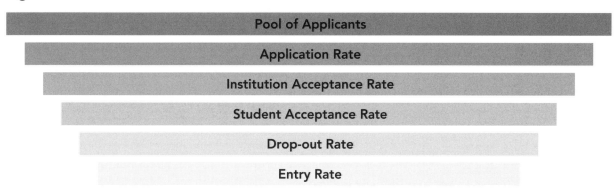

In this framework, the number of candidates who complete their training and enter the workforce is determined by a series of six major filters that can be hierarchically grouped into a "funnel". Figure 6 depicts this "funnel" and its six filters: the pool of potential applicants (i.e. the number of people who are eligible to apply for a certain educational track to become a health-worker; the application rate (i.e. the proportion of people applying to a health educational track to become a health worker, among all eligible people); the institution acceptance rate (i.e. the proportion of people accepted into a specific educational track to become a health worker, among those who apply); the student acceptance rate (i.e. the proportion of people who accept an educational place, among those who have been accepted); the success rate (i.e. the proportion of people who graduate from an educational track, among those who entered it); and the entry rate (i.e. the proportion of people who join the health workforce, among those who complete their education).

These rates may be determined by a number of factors both within and outside a planner's control. The pool of applicants and application rate, for example, may be fundamentally constrained by the levels and quality of the country's secondary education. In contrast, the institutional acceptance rate can be regulated by the institutions themselves (e.g. limiting the number of medical school places), and the drop-out rate has been shown to be affected by choice of pedagogical method. The evidence base surrounding each of these filters is discussed further in Annex 3.

Quality of graduates

The education funnel determines the level of the health workforce in a country and, if stratified by certain characteristics, such as gender, place of birth, or employment sector, can be used to assess the influence of education on the distribution of health workers. But education also plays an important role in shaping the clinical as well as the service quality of the health workforce, i.e. the performance of health workers. While content selection and the quality of teachers and teaching methods influence the knowledge, skills and attitudes of students, trainees or residents, there has been a worldwide trend in education for the health professions to emphasize academic knowledge over the skills needed to work in clinical settings (Majoor, 2004). In many African countries, for example, medical curricula often reflect the health trends and capacities of industrialized countries, while neglecting to teach the knowledge, skills and attitudes vital for local health care, for example how to treat diseases that are priorities for developing countries, understanding the relationship between scientific and traditional medicine, the realities of rural health care in the field, and health care management in circumstances of resource constraints and uncertainty (Ndumbe, 2003; Majoor, 2004). In some countries, fields of health care which are important in the context of prevalent diseases and available resources (e.g. public health) are not taught at all.

A number of frameworks have been proposed to assess the quality of health professionals education. Among them, the World Federation for Medical Education (WFME) standards (WFME, 2003) were chosen as a starting point for identifying indicators of the quality of health professionals education. WFME identifies nine areas of quality assessment and potential improvement of health professionals education:

- mission and objectives
- educational programme
- assessment of students
- students
- academic staff
- educational resources
- programme evaluation
- governance and administration
- continuous renewal.

The WFME framework was chosen rather than the other frameworks that were reviewed because:

- it was more comprehensive in its coverage of areas of educational quality;
- it was more detailed in its suggestions for indicators of educational quality;
- its indicators seemed more practicable to implement globally (the WFME tool was developed for all countries worldwide, while other tools were usually developed for application in one specific country).

Annex 3 gives an overview of alternative frameworks that could be used to assess the quality of education of human resources for health.

While the basic structure of the WFME (2003) document (i.e. nine areas in which quality should be assessed) is followed, various changes were made in order to adapt the framework and its derived indicators to the purpose of this tool. These changes include:

- addition (or deletion) of sub-areas to (or from) the list of sub-areas of educational quality proposed by WFME (2001);
- addition (or deletion) of indicators to (or from) the list of indicators to assess educational quality proposed by WFME (2001);
- operationalization of certain areas of quality into indicators;
- prioritization of indicators (into primary and secondary indicators).

These changes were necessary because the focus of the WFME (2003) document is basic medical education, while this tool needs to be able to assess education of all health workers, i.e. including nursing education, post-graduate medical education, community health worker education, etc. In addition, many of the indicators in WFME (2003) document are descriptions of existing structures, processes, or activities, but do not lend themselves to benchmarking exercises.

Depending on the context of the assessment at hand (task definition, resources available for the assessment, etc.) the analyst will need to use the indicators in different ways, including assessing the indicators at country level (for instance, if national policies define the structure and process of health professionals education) or assessing the indicators in a representative sample of educational institutions for health workers (for instance, if educational institutions are able to define large proportions of their curricula independently).

The core indicators for assessing the quality of the education of the health workforce are given in the following table.

Table 6. Education of human resources for health (HRH): primary indicators

Dimension	Indicator	Bench-mark	Reference	Comments	
				Indicator/ benchmark	Source
• HRH level: pool of potential applicants	% second-ary schooling attainment or % second-ary schooling enrolment	91 (net enrolment in high income countries) 74 (gross enrolment in middle income countries) 44 (gross enrolment in low income countries)	*Benchmark:* • (World Bank, 2004)	Further indicators: • number of graduating middle school students (aggregate and by distribution dimensions) • number of graduating high school students (aggregate and by distribution dimensions) • number of graduating medical school students (aggregate and by distribution dimensions) • proportion of applicants to health professions educational institutions who are not same year graduates of an educational programme qualifying for an application to a health professions educational institution (aggregate and by distribution dimensions) *Comment:* In some countries, for instance in countries with mandatory military service for men, this proportion may be quite high. However, as long as the proportion does not change much over time, the numbers of graduating students will be a good approximation of the total pool of potential applicants.	Can be assessed through ministry of education documents

Dimension	Indicator	Bench-mark	Reference	Comments	
				Indicator/ benchmark	Source
• HRH level: application rate	Number of applicants per HRH educa-tion place	1.9 (USA) 1.5 (mini-mum)	*Benchmark:* • (Cooper, 2003)	Further indicators: • proportion of high school graduates (aggregate and by distribution dimensions) applying to: – medical schools – public health schools – pharmaceutical schools – nursing and midwifery schools – health assistant and para-medical training schools • proportion of middle school graduates (aggregate and by distribution dimen-sions) applying to: – nursing and midwifery schools – health assistant and paramedical training • proportion of medical school graduates (aggre-gate and by distribution dimensions) applying for residency training, by specialization category Determinants of application rate: • proportion of middle and high school graduates reached by HRH infor-mation and promotion campaigns • average cost of education, by HRH education track Constraints to application rate: • average annual earning, by HRH category • average hourly salaries, by HRH category • rank in surveys of "most admired occupation" • proportion of HRH, by category, who are currently unemployed • Average annual earning, by HRH category	Can be assessed through: ministry of education documents, HRH education insti-tution documents or interviews with HRH school administrators

Dimension	Indicator	Bench-mark	Reference	Comments	
				Indicator/ benchmark	Source
• HRH level: institutional acceptance rate	Proportion of applicants (aggregate and by distribution dimensions) accepted into a specific type of HRH education institution	None	None	Determinants of the institutional acceptance rate: • number of places, by HRH education track Constraints to the institutional acceptance rate: • distribution of grade point averages of students applying to HRH education	
• HRH level: applicant acceptance rate	Proportion of applicants accepting HRH education place	Close to 100%	*Benchmark:* • Ideal	Constraint to the institutional acceptance rate: • proportion of applicants (aggregate and by distribution dimensions) applying to more than one school (by HRH education track)	Can be assessed through ministry of education documents, HRH education institution documents or interviews with HRH school administrators
• HRH level: HRH education success rate	Graduates (aggregate and by distribution dimensions) as proportion of all original entrants	85% in medical schools (South Africa) 90%–95% nursing schools (South Africa)	*Benchmark:* • (Huddart & Picazo, 2003)	Determinants of success rate: • reasons for drop-out as perceived by: – drop-outs – successful students – HRH educators	Can be assessed through ministry of education documents, HRH education institution documents or interviews with HRH school administrators
• HRH level: entry rate	Proportion of graduates entering the health sector	Close to 100%	*Benchmark:* • Ideal	Can be divided into a public and private sector entry rate. Further information: • reasons for non-entry as perceived by graduates who do not enter • focus of HRH curricula on national priority diseases and not on diseases of little relevance in the country context	Can be assessed through ministry of education documents, ministry of health
• HRH distribution: geographic distribution	Highest-to-lowest regional graduate density	None	None		Can be assessed through ministry of education documents, ministry of health
• HRH distribution: gender distribution	Proportion of HRH graduates who are female	50%	*Benchmark:* • Equity rationale	Will usually need to be assessed for each HRH category separately	Can be assessed through ministry of education and ministry of health documents

33

Dimension	Indicator	Bench-mark	Reference	Comments	
				Indicator/ benchmark	Source
• HRH per-formance: mission and objectives (statements)	Inclusion in mission statement of readiness for health care work or further training, social responsibility, research and community involvement	Existence	*Indicator:* • WFME (2003) (adapted)		Can be assessed through document re-view or key informant interviews at HRH education institutions
• HRH per-formance: educational programme (clinical sciences and skills)	Student par-ticipation in patient care	Number of hours spent in patient care per week	*Indicator:* • WFME (2003) (adapted)		Can be assessed through document re-view or key informant interviews at HRH education institutions or observation of clinical care
• HRH per-formance: educational programme (clinical sciences and skills)	Proportion of courses devoted to country prior-ity diseases	None	None	For example,courses on HIV, malaria, tuberculosis, etc.	Can be assessed through HRH educa-tional institutions
• HRH per-formance: students (student intake)	Size of the student intake defined in rela-tionship to the capacity of the HRH educa-tion institution at all stages of the education	None	*Indicator:* • WFME (2003)	Further information: • Are mechanisms in place to regularly update the student intake as capacity changes?	Can be assessed through key infor-mant interviews at HRH education institutions
• HRH per-formance: assessment of students (service quality)	Admission policy	Existence	*Indicator:* • WFME (2003)		Can be assessed through document review
• HRH per-formance: academic staff (staff policy and develop-ment)	Mechanisms for upgrading of teaching skills	Existence	*Indicator:* • WFME (2003) (adapted)		Can be assessed through document review, key informant interviews at HRH education institutions

Dimension	Indicator	Bench-mark	Reference	Comments	
				Indicator/ benchmark	Source
• HRH performance: educational resources (teacher input intensity)	Average classroom size	None	None		Can be assessed through ministry of education documents, HRH education institution documents or interviews with HRH school administrators
• HRH performance: educational resources (computer access)	Number of computers per student				Can be assessed through document review, key informant interviews at HRH education institutions or inspection tours
• HRH performance: educational resources (Internet access)	Number of computers with Internet access per student				Can be assessed through document review or key informant interviews at HRH education institutions or inspection tours
• HRH performance: programme evaluation (stakeholder involvement)	Stakeholder involvement in programme evaluation	Yes	*Indicator:* • WFME (2003) (adapted)	The principal stakeholders of the specific HRH education track need to be defined first	Can be assessed through document review or key informant interviews at HRH education institutions
• HRH performance: governance and administration (governance)	Defined governance structures	Existence	*Indicator:* WFME (2003) (adapted)	Further information: • Do governance structures reflect representation from academic staff, students and other stakeholders?	Can be assessed through document review or key informant interviews at HRH education institutions
• HRH performance: governance and administration (academic leadership)	Clear lines of responsibility and authority for the curriculum and the educational budget	Existence	*Indicator:* WFME (2003) (adapted)		Can be assessed through document review or key informant interviews at HRH education institutions
• HRH performance: continuous renewal	Mechanisms for regular review of HRH education	Existence	*Indicator:* WFME (2003) (adapted)	The review should include: • educational mission • curriculum • instructional methods • assessment methods	Can be assessed through document review or key informant interviews at HRH education institutions

MANAGEMENT

Just as the performance of the health sector is largely dependent upon health worker performance, system performance requires effective management of human resources (Martineau & Martinez, 1997; Buchan, 2004). Though this "growing body" of evidence suggests that "good" or "high commitment" human resources management is associated with better performance (Buchan, 2004), just what those practices are – and how performance is measured – is not always so clear or consistently measured (Gould-Williams, 2004). Furthermore, health workforce policies are not implemented in a vacuum, and there is evidence that environmental factors such as working conditions, organizational climate and internal consistency of health systems influence the effectiveness of management practices related to human resources (Rondeau & Wagar, 2001; Green & Collins, 2003; Buchan, 2004).

This section of the tool suggests methods for assessing the management capacities and conditions which govern human resources. Assessments of human resources have traditionally emphasized workforce numbers, skills and distribution. In the context of the public sector or of developing countries, this has translated into a focus on human resources management or human resources development, usually revolving around the administrative capacities to implement an array of systems, policies and practices governing personnel concerns. Components typically associated with human resources management or human resources development include a variety of personnel management practices, including personnel policies (e.g. job classification systems, compensation and benefits, recruitment, transfers, promotion, discipline or grievance procedures, and personnel files) (MSH, 1998).

The term "management" is, however, interpreted more broadly in the context of this tool: it encompasses not only the management *of* human resources, but management *by* human resources of processes at various levels of the system. Such thinking is in line with more recent assessments of human resources for health, which are concerned with management matters related to public versus private provision of services, civil service reform, logistics management, performance management, and staff retention (Van Lerberghe et al., 2002a; Ferlie & Shortell, 2001). Thus internal channels of communication which can have an effect on the performance of managers are assessed alongside capacities to administer personnel-related files; and rules that regulate decisions from the central to the peripheral level are considered to influence management as much as facility-level management culture.

The framework used here for management assessment is outlined in Figure 7. The following sections describe in greater detail the hypothesized links between each element of management and the health workforce outcomes, as well as suggesting indicators for analysis of a country's particular management situation. It should be noted that indicators in this section are often imperfect proxies for complex management concepts and that subjective judgments by management experts should accompany any quantitative indicators.

Figure 7. Rapid assessment of management of human resources for health (HRH)

Public sector context • Decentralization of human resources functions • Other specific initiatives on human resources	**MACRO**
Stewardship of HRH • Senior management of public sector HRH • Engagement with the private and NGO sector	
Core administration of human resources management [5] • Job descriptions, performance review • Career path (job classification system, promotion) • HRH deployment (recruitment, transfer, discipline, grievances, termination) • Personnel files • Health management information system	**MESO**
Institutional environment • Working conditions (adequate supplies, equipment) • Intra-system communication	**MICRO**
Facility organizational practices • Teamwork • Vision, high standards, clear expectations	

Public sector context

Ministries of health are often bound by conditions which affect all public sector employees, not just those in the health sector. As such, rules, regulations and reforms within the public sector affect both the health system's capacity to manage human resources, as well as the capacity of health workers to manage their designated functions. Governmental decentralization, for example, may constrain or enable the ability of local-level managers to hire, fire, transfer, pay and promote staff. This, in turn, will have a huge effect on health system performance (Kolehmainen-Aitken, 2004). Since there is no reason to believe that civil service reform or decentralization will automatically lead to improved human resources management and system performance (Bossert & Beauvais, 2002; Van Lerberghe et al., 2002b; Bossert et al., 2003), an understanding of both of these elements is important in analysing the macro-level environment which shapes management of and by health workers. Indeed, the evidence base suggests that the link between the public sector context and system performance is complex (see Annex 4 for further discussion on the evidence base).

Additional policies which apply across the public sector but are not related to decentralization may also affect management capacities and human resources for health. A country's government, for instance, might require individual ministries to develop and implement sector-specific human resource development policies. As with decentralization-related issues, awareness of such policies can aid in understanding how the public sector context influences management concerns. The core indicators for assessing the management of human resources for health in the public sector are given in the following table.

---

[5] The assessment of compensation and benefits systems is addressed in the section on financing.

Table 7. Management of human resources for health (HRH): primary indicators for the public sector context

Dimension	Indicator	Bench-mark	Reference	Comments	
				Indicator/ Benchmark	Sources
• Decentralization	Choice over salary range (narrow, moderate, wide)	None	*Indicator:* • Bossert (1998) (adapted)	Narrow: determined by law or authority higher than ministry of health Moderate: multiple models for local choice (e.g. national *minimum* standards; flexibility in job classification) Wide: no limits	Can be assessed through document review or key informant interviews
• Decentralization	Ability to hire/fire (narrow, moderate, wide)	None	*Indicator:* • Bossert (1998) (adapted)	Narrow: determined by national civil service rules Moderate: determined by local civil service rules Wide: determined by no civil service rules	Can be assessed through document review or key informant interviews
• Decentralization	Choice over staff deployment or facility staffing norms (narrow, moderate, wide)	None	*Indicator:* • Bossert (1998) (adapted)	Narrow: determined by ministry of health at central level Moderate: multiple models for local choice (e.g. national *minimum* standards; multiple or equivalent staffing patterns allowed) Wide: no super-local standards	Can be assessed through document review or key informant interviews
• Decentralization	Choice over staff recruitment (narrow, moderate, wide)	None	*Indicator:* • Bossert (1998) (adapted)	Narrow: determined by ministry of health at central level Moderate: multiple models for local choice Wide: no super-local standards	Can be assessed through document review or key informant interviews
• Decentralization	Choice over staff transfers (narrow, moderate, wide)	None	*Indicator:* • Bossert (1998) (adapted)	Narrow: determined by ministry of health at central level Moderate: multiple models for local choice Wide: no super-local standards	Can be assessed through document review or key informant interviews
• Decentralization	Choice over staff promotion (narrow, moderate, wide)	None	*Indicator:* • Bossert (1998) (adapted)	Narrow: determined by ministry of health at central level Moderate: multiple models for local choice Wide: no super-local standards	Can be assessed through document review or key informant interviews
• Decentralization	Choice over resource allocation (% local spending explicitly earmarked by higher authorities)	None	*Indicator:* • Bossert (1998) (adapted)	Narrow: high % Moderate: mid % Wide: low %	Can be assessed through document review or key informant interviews
• Other specific initiatives on human resources	Existence of public sector-wide initiatives relating to human resources	None			Can be assessed through document review or key informant interviews

Stewardship of the health workforce

The concept of governmental stewardship of a health system extends to the context of human resources for health. As described in *The world health report 2000* (WHO, 2000), an effective health system steward (i.e. a country's ministry of health) will help attain health system goals by ensuring acceptable quality and coverage of health services in both the public and private sectors. In terms of public sector services, stewardship revolves around direct organization and management of the health care system. Outside the public sector, a ministry of health is expected to use such indirect tools as oversight and private sector engagement. These two sets of stewardship skills apply to human resources for health as well.

In terms of direct organization and management of human resources for health, top-level commitment to rational management activities is likely to be an important component. It is true that decentralization or increased sub-national decision-making power may provide lower-level managers with space to effectively implement human resources management or human resources development activities. However, total abdication of central-level involvement could also increase fragmentation and inhibit effective management and planning practices in the system. Thus, leadership capable of motivating workers to work towards better human resources management and development may be especially important (Franco et al., 2002; Green & Collins, 2003).

Even if national-level commitment to human resources management and development does exist, an overly-downsized central ministry may inhibit effective management of the health workforce simply for lack of sufficient personnel. Both commitment by staff and the capacities of key players at each level of the system, including their capacity to recruit staff, are important in establishing an environment conducive to effective management. As an example, management training is increasingly recognized as an important determinant of health workers' performance. High-level support which can link such training with human resources management or development policies, particularly in the context of decentralized decision-making authority, may thus be important in ensuring appropriately trained managers. Though few studies analyse leadership and system outcomes at this level, there is some evidence that such commitment is associated with positive organizational outcomes (see Annex 4 for further discussion on the evidence base).

In terms of engagement with the private sector, stewardship involves policies and regulations which either promote or restrict practices related to human resources for health. An actively updated registration system for different cadres of health workers is a prerequisite for governmental enforcement of regulatory mechanisms governing the private sector. Examples of the latter include clearly articulated regulations regarding multiple job holding (it is not uncommon for the public sector to ignore this practice through lack of regulatory legislation) and spelling out modes of contracting for health services with the private sector. The core indicators for assessing the effectiveness of stewardship of human resources for health are given in the following table.

Table 8. Management of human resources for health (HRH): primary indicators for stewardship of HRH

Dimension	Indicator	Bench-mark	Reference	Comments	
				Indicator/benchmark	Source
• Senior management of HRH	% budget allocated to HRM or HRD annually	None	*Indicator:* • MSH (1998) (adapted)	*Indicator:* Effective HRM or HRD not possible without financial resources	Can be assessed through review of ministry of health budget documents
• Senior management of HRH	Number of full-time equivalent high-level HRM or HRD staff	1+ according to need	*Indicator:* • MSH (1998) (adapted) *Benchmark:* • MSH (1998)	*Indicator:* Effective HRM or HRD requires top-level direction (World Bank, 2003). *Benchmark:* While HRD or HRM responsibilities may be divided between several persons, coherent programmes and policies may be more difficult to achieve	Can be assessed through review of ministry of health personnel documents or key informant interviews at national level

Dimension	Indicator	Bench-mark	Reference	Comments	
				Indicator/benchmark	Source
• Senior management of HRH	Ratio of central level managers to regional level managers	None		*Indicator:* Adequate numbers of central level staff must be available to provide system management, including HRM and HRD; too low a ratio may indicate insufficient personnel to direct health sector development.	Can be assessed through review of ministry of health management information system documents
• Senior management of HRH	Documented HRM or HRD plan exists	Yes	*Indicator:* • MSH (1998) (adapted) *Benchmark:* • MSH (1998)	*Indicator:* Effective HRM and HRD require top-level direction – a documented plan is one element of such direction	Can be assessed through review of ministry of health strategic planning documents or key informant interviews at national level
• Senior management of HRH	% staff at various levels receiving management training in past year	None	•	*Indicator:* ongoing programme of skills updating is necessary for effective HRM and HRD	Can be assessed through review of ministry of health budget documents
• Senior management of HRH	Mission statement or goals linked to HRM or HRD planning	Yes	*Indicator:* • MSH (1998) (adapted) *Benchmark:* • MSH (1998)	*Indicator:* effective HRM or HRD requires top-level direction – actively linking documented HRM or HRD plan with mission goals is one element of such direction	Can be assessed through review of ministry of health strategic planning documents or key informant interviews at national or subnational level
• Private sector engagement	Private provider registration system is up to date and accurate	Yes		Effective interaction with or regulation of the private sector requires accurate knowledge of the numbers, types and qualifications of private sector providers	Can be assessed through document review or key informant interviews
• Private sector engagement	Number of provider contracting models allowed	None	*Indicator:* (Bossert, 1998) (adapted)	Narrow: none or 1 Moderate: several specified Wide: no limits	Can be assessed through document review or key informant interviews
• Private sector engagement	Number of public sector health workforce categories permitted to work at least part-time in private sector	None	*Indicator:* • this tool	Restrictions on categories of public sector workers (e.g. physicians, pharmacists, nurses) permitted to work at least part-time in the private sector can affect facility-level relations with private sector providers	Can be assessed through document review

Human resources management

The performance of the health workforce depends greatly on the core administrative components (Figure 7) of human resources management being effectively managed. Well-formulated job descriptions, for instance, reflect good organizational and management competencies, are a prerequisite for performance review, and can be an important element in improving management training and practices (Ruck et al., 1999). A well-defined career path may be an important component in attracting and retaining employees, yet such structures often exist only for doctors and nurses (Martinez & Martineau, 1998). Other aspects, such as up-to-date and comprehensive personnel and payroll files are also felt to be indicative of adequate management competence (World Bank, 2003), though no studies could be found specifically relating those elements to performance. Finally, effective use of health management information systems can fundamentally affect the way in which an organization operates and the efficiency of its management of personnel (Helfenbein et al., 1987). Conversely, a poorly run health management information system is an indicator of underlying managerial deficiencies in using data for decisions (Lippeveld et al., 2000).

No information relating other core administrative aspects of human resources management – such as policy manuals or orientation programmes – to human resources outcomes or performance could be found in the literature. Though few studies have isolated the links between each of those elements and health workforce or systems performance, there is some indication that they are collectively important in better functioning systems (see Annex 4 for further discussion on the evidence base). The core indicators for assessing the administration of human resources for health are given in the following table.

Table 9. Management of human resources for health (HRH): primary indicators for core administrative components of human resources management (HRM)

Dimension	Indicator	Bench-mark	Reference	Comments	
				Indicator/ Benchmark	Sources
• Adequate over-all management system	Master file exists which contains records of employee history, job descriptions, etc.	Yes	*Indicator:* • World Bank (2003) (adapted) *Benchmark:* • World Bank (2003)	While personnel information may exist across several file or record-keeping systems, a reliable, complete, current and definitive source of information (i.e. a master file) is necessary	Can be assessed through document review, or key informant interviews at national or sub-national levels
• Adequate over-all management system	Guidelines exist for accessing personnel files	Yes	*Indicator:* • World Bank (2003) (adapted) *Benchmark:* • World Bank (2003)	Guidelines cannot be effective unless they are accessible	Can be assessed through document review, or key informant interviews at national or sub-national levels
• Adequate over-all management system	Policy manual exists to aid personnel administration	Yes	*Indicator:* • World Bank (2003) (adapted) *Benchmark:* • World Bank (2003)	Records management procedures need to be documented for operations and training	Can be assessed through document review, or key informant interviews at national or sub-national levels
• Performance appraisal	Performance appraisal guidelines documented and accessible	Yes	*Indicator:* • World Bank (2003) (adapted) *Benchmark:* • Ideal	Performance appraisal is an important part of personnel administration, and accessible, accurate and up-to-date guidelines are necessary for guidelines to be effective	Can be assessed through document review, or key informant interviews at national or sub-national levels

Dimension	Indicator	Bench-mark	Reference	Comments	
				Indicator/ Benchmark	Sources
• Career path	Job classification system identifies families of jobs with distinct skills and evolution of promotion (high, medium, low)	High	*Indicator:* • World Bank (2003) (adapted) *Benchmark:* • Ideal	Clearly documented career path progression is necessary for effective personnel management	Can be assessed through document review, or key informant interviews at national or subnational levels
• HRH deployment	Guidelines exist for forms and procedures for approving recruitment, promotions and transfers	Yes	*Indicator:* • World Bank (2003) (adapted) *Benchmark:* • Ideal	Clearly documented career path progression is necessary for effective personnel management	Can be assessed through document review or key informant interviews at national or subnational levels
• HRH deployment	Guidelines exist for forms and procedures for discipline, grievances and termination	Yes	*Indicator:* • World Bank (2003) (adapted) *Benchmark:* • Ideal	Clearly documented career path progression is necessary for effective personnel management	Can be assessed through document review, or key informant interviews at national or sub-national levels
• Personnel files	Recruitment, promotions and transfer records checked against authorized posts, annual budgets and available funds	Yes	*Indicator:* • World Bank (2003) (adapted) *Benchmark:* • Ideal	A link between health workforce deployment and salary levels, and between budget and strategic plans, is necessary for efficient systems management	Can be assessed through document review, or key informant interviews at national or subnational levels
• Health management information system	Number of times per year the health management information system provides feedback on indicator reporting	At least once per year or on a regular basis	*Benchmark:* • Best practices	Feedback from higher levels of the system to lower levels is important in facilitating intra-level communication and system performance assessment	Can be assessed through review of strategic planning, and quarterly and annual documents, or key informant interviews
• Health management information system	% facilities using current indicator forms for monitoring & evaluation reporting (e.g. morbidity reports)	100%	*Indicator:* • World Bank (2003) (adapted) *Benchmark:* • Ideal	Assessment of capacity of lower level facilities to provide or use information corresponding to the ministry of health's priorities or needs	Can be assessed through internationally-accessible databases, in-country databases and ministry of health documents, or by panel of experts or other methods of estimation
• Health management information system	% facilities submitting disease notifications as required	100%	*Indicator:* • World Bank (2003) (adapted) *Benchmark:* • Ideal	Assessment of capacity of lower-level facilities to provide or use information corresponding to the ministry of health's priorities or needs	Can be assessed through internationally-accessible databases, in-country databases and ministry of health documents

Institutional environment

The environment within which health workers operate, as well as the relationship which they have with their working environment, may affect outcomes in several ways. Satisfactory or enabling working conditions are prerequisites for personnel performance. A poor working environment can be a main reason for heightened workplace distress and decreased job satisfaction (Bodur, 2002). In contrast, an adequate stock of supplies, functioning equipment and a manageable workload can directly improve the quality of care. Yet these elements are often lacking in developing countries: primary and secondary health care facilities often lack such basic supplies and equipment as essential medicines and beds (Barua et al., 2003; Simoes et al., 2003).

Extreme levels of staff rotation – either excessively high or excessively low rates – among certain health professions may lead to negative consequences, including an inability to carry out management change, higher costs of recruiting and training, and disruption of social and communication structures (Koh & Goh, 1995; Collins et al., 2000).

Effective communication between levels of a health system is an important mechanism to ensure efficient and rational provision of services to patients as well. For example, communication between different categories of health workers has been linked to better performance in developed-country hospital settings (Scott et al., 2003a), and a well-functioning referral system is considered to be the centrepiece of a primary health care approach to service delivery which emphasizes just such communication (WHO & UNICEF, 1978). Again, however, these elements are often not in place. For instance, extremely low rates of clinic-to-hospital referral (less than 2% of all patients) are the norm in many parts of the world, particularly sub-Saharan Africa (Nordberg et al., 1996; Font et al., 2002).

The core indicators for assessing institutional relations in the context of the management of the health workforce are given in the following table. For further discussion on empirical evidence linking the institutional environment and institutional relations to performance, see Annex 4.

Table 10. Management of human resources for health (HRH): primary indicators of institutional environment

Dimension	Indicator	Benchmark	Reference	Comments	
				Indicator/benchmark	Source
• Working conditions	Stockouts of essential medicines	0%	*Indicator:* • DELIVER/ John Snow (2002) (adapted) *Benchmark:* • Ideal	Indicator of system-level management capacities which affect facility-level performance	Can be assessed through document review (e.g. national drug policy and pharmaceutical management study) or key informant interviews
• Working conditions	% difference between stock on hand and stock recorded in inventory system	0%	*Indicator:* • DELIVER/ John Snow (2002) (adapted) *Benchmark:* • Ideal	Indicator of system-level management capacities which affect facility-level performance	Can be assessed through document review (e.g. national drug policy and pharmaceutical management study) or key informant interviews
• Working conditions	% facilities with acceptable storage facilities (adequate shelving, refrigeration, electricity)	100%	*Indicator:* • DELIVER/ John Snow (2002) (adapted) *Benchmark:* • Ideal	Indicator of system-level management capacities which affect facility-level performance	Can be assessed through document review (e.g. national drug policy and pharmaceutical management study) or key informant interviews

Dimension	Indicator	Bench-mark	Reference	Comments	
				Indicator/ benchmark	Source
• Workload statutary	Number of hours actually worked per number of working hours	1	*Indicator:* • Hornby & Forte (2000) *Benchmark:* • Ideal	Indicates degree of work overload	Can be assessed through review of service statistics or key informant interviews
• Intra-level communication, in service supervision	Number and frequency of supervisory visits to health post or health centre facilities	At least one/ per year or on regular basis	*Benchmark:* • Best prac-tices	Regular supervision and oversight from higher levels of the system to lower levels is important in facilitating intra-level communication and sys-tem performance	Ideally assessed through service statistics or quantita-tive survey; can also be assessed through key informant interviews
• Staff rotation	Annual number of job leavers per average staff in post + leavers	None cur-rently avail-able	*Indicator:* • Hornby & Forte (2000)		Can be assessed through internation-ally-accessible data-bases, in-country da-tabases and ministry of health documents, or by panel of experts or other methods of estimation

Facility organizational practices

By shaping the environment which frames day-to-day actions, such facility-level practices as organizational culture and leadership at the facility level affect personnel performance. While no precise definition or consensus on the exact nature of organizational culture exists, the term is usually used to denote a wide range of social processes within an institution which help "define an organization's character and norms" (Scott et al., 2003b).

Organizational culture in the health care setting is often measured quantitatively through in-depth studies (e.g. 15 – 120 questions in length). Categorizations of organizational culture are either typological (e.g. hierarchy versus market type) or dimensional (e.g. supervision, staff attitudes, benefits, cohesiveness) (Scott et al., 2003b). Leadership in the health sector shares many of the characteristics of organizational culture. Leadership has been variously defined as "the capacity of individuals to influence others toward the accomplishment of organizationally relevant goals/objectives" or as "an ongoing conversation among people who care deeply about something of great importance" (Shortell et al., 1991; Ferlie & Shortell, 2001). Leadership, too, is usually measured with lengthy surveys (Huber et al., 2000). And various typologies of leadership exist, from transactional and transformational to contingent and situational (Bass & Avolio, 1990; Clark & Clark, 1990; Hersey et al., 2001).

Based on earlier research findings, this tool suggests indicators on two aspects of organizational culture and leadership, hypothesized to be determinants of health workforce outcomes.[6] The first aspect comprises teamwork and participatory decision-making. The second covers vision, high standards, and clear expectations. Both sets of factors have been linked to better organizational and system outcomes (see Annex 4 for further discussion on the evidence base). The core indicators for assessing organizational practices in health facilities are given in the table below.

---

[6] An in-depth study of organizational culture and leadership which could definitively link those determinants to health workforce out-comes is beyond the scope of this tool. However, Annex 4 provides examples of possible research instruments should the consultant team have the time and resources to implement a study of leadership or organizational culture.

Table 11. Management of human resources for health (HRH): primary indicators of facility organizational practices

Dimension	Indicator	Bench-mark	Reference	Comments	
				Indicator/ benchmark	Source
Teamwork, participatory decision-making	Frequency or number of staff meetings per year	At least one per quarter		Frequent and regular staff meetings are important for effective facility-level management of HRH	Can be assessed through document review (e.g. quarterly reports) and key informant interviews
• Vision, high standards, and clear expectations	% staff meeting agendas per minutes documented	100%	*Indicator:* • Diaz-Monsalve (2004) *Benchmark:* • Ideal	Indicates whether structure of meetings is adequately managed	Can be assessed through document review (e.g. quarterly reports) and key informant interviews
• Management capacity	Management training modules offered regularly to managers on pre-service or in-service basis	Yes	*Indicator:* • MSH (1998) (adapted) *Benchmark:* • Ideal	Indicates management competencies	Can be assessed through document review (e.g. quarterly reports) and key informant interviews

POLICY-MAKING FOR HUMAN RESOURCES FOR HEALTH

Making any type of change within the health sector involves a political process. *The world health report 2000* emphasizes the need for political and stakeholder analysis in assessing health system performance – two aspects of performance that were missing from previous analyses (WHO, 2000). This section outlines one method of assessing the political context of human resources for health, and of developing strategies for gaining support for policies in the area of human resources for health.

We suggest following the framework for analysis of policy-making using a stakeholder analysis based on a software package entitled *Policymaker* (Reich, 1996). The framework identifies five main steps to be taken to conduct a proper stakeholder analysis for assessing policy-making processes, and for developing and evaluating political strategies for influencing policy:

- *Policy.* Define and analyse the contents of the policy changes and reforms that are selected to address the problems identified. This includes identifying both the goals of the policies and the mechanisms or specific policies needed to achieve these goals.
- *Players.* Identify all key players (stakeholders) that may be involved in the field of human resources for health. Determine their positions, power and interests, and the consequences of the policy for each player. Networks and coalitions should be examined as well.
- *Opportunities and obstacles.* Analyse the contextual opportunities and obstacles that might affect whether the policy or reform will be adopted and implemented.
- *Strategies.* Define political strategies that can be used to achieve adoption and implementation of the policy or reform. These strategies may involve a variety of advocacy tools to mobilize key supporting stakeholders and reduce opposition.
- *Impacts.* Estimate how each of the strategies will affect the future position and power of the players. This estimate will produce an assessment of the feasibility of achieving adoption and implementation of the policy or reform and may lead to an action plan.

The literature relating human resources for health to politics and policy is limited. In some countries that have implemented health workforce reforms, a number of case studies have investigated the policy environments and reform strategies. However, there is little empirical evidence concerning which political environment is best for human resources for health. The following section discusses the different aspects of the general political environment that should be investigated as the assessment team develops policy proposals for changes in the financing, education and management of human resources for health. We recommend that the assessment team develop a careful stakeholder analysis through interviews with key stakeholders and with academic or other observers with experience in political analysis and knowledge of the health sector. The following section is a brief introduction to the key areas for analysis, and provides a general overview of possible stakeholder positions and power.

Policy context

In order to define the appropriate policy for human resources for health in a country, background research must be conducted to develop a picture of the general political system of the country. This analysis should include the type of government system in place, the general ability of the State to enforce laws and regulations, the basic procedures and processes of government.

Type of government system in place

The feasibility of different strategies for changing policies related to human resources for health will be influenced by the type of regime that is in place. The types of reforms that can be adopted, the stakeholders who participate in the policy process, and the types of strategies which will be effective in building support for policy changes will be influenced by the degree and pervasiveness of democratic instititions in a country. In many democratic countries, for instance, unions can be significant political actors in promoting health workforce policies and popular demands can be influential. Countries with less democratic institutions, however, usually exclude unions from the policy process and may be more responsive to interests of specific elites than the populace. The role of party politics also varies by type of governments, with some systems requiring the support of political parties for reforms and others relying more on strong interest groups. While there are no hard and fast rules regarding constraints that governments place on political feasibility of reform, it is important to assess this characteristic as a context for developing a political strategy for reforms.

Laws and regulation

Implementing a successful policy change is not easy, since it involves multiple steps and actors. The State's capability to enforce laws and regulations will therefore be essential to carrying out any type of policy. An assessment of the country's ability to enforce laws should be conducted and should include such elements as current regulations on private practice, licensing of physicians and other health workers, and accreditation of hospitals and other health facilities. If the government does not have a positive record of enforcing laws and regulations, changing a health workforce policy could be a challenge.

Process of policy change

Identifying the history of policy change in the health sector in a country involves a close examination of the history of health policies and the role of stakeholders in that process. For example, in some countries the role of professional associations is paramount, while in others these associations have not been effectively organized for policy issues. In some countries, a dominant political party will have a history of promoting progressive legislation, while in others the main party will be more conservative and oriented towards the status quo.

Corruption

Assessing the policy environment also includes identifying barriers to policy change such as corruption. Corruption is often hard to eliminate once in place, and may have to be considered a contextual factor in the political process (Klitgaard, 2000). For instance, if the health workforce policy involves increasing or decreasing salaries or changing the positions of certain medical personnel, corruption could hinder these reforms. In some civil service reforms, it has been found that raising salaries decreases the prevalence of bribes, but increases their monetary size (Rose-Ackerman, 1997). Although ending corruption in a country may be difficult, it will be important to at least identify the magnitude of corruption in order to adjust policies accordingly.

Transparency

Transparency may also be an important ingredient for health workforce policy change. Access to information on the health workforce and on how new policies will help the country may assist in policy advocacy. Restrictions on information or lack of credibility of official data may protect stakeholders who are advantaged by the status quo and limit the effectiveness of policy design and the likelihood of gaining support for policy reforms.

Players, position, and power

One of the key tasks in stakeholder analysis is to determine the position that different actors will take on the specific human resource policy reform that the assessment proposes. It is important to analyse the actors' positions vis-à-vis specific proposals, because these positions may change depending on the content of the proposal. It is also important to recognize that many of the potential proposals are likely to generate significant opposition from stakeholders who generally benefit from the existing system. Reforms may threaten the interests of different groups of health workers and demand reallocation of resources from other sectors. Often the beneficiaries (e.g. the new health workers or the populations to be served by new workers) are not aware or not yet mobilized to support the reforms.

In addition, the power of actors is difficult to assess. Power may be based on tangible factors such as money, votes or organizational capacities, or on intangible resources such as control of information, credibility and access to policy-makers. This section suggests a range of power (high, medium, low) for each of the major actors discussed above. Usually the highest power stakeholders include the president, ministry of finance, ministry of planning, ministry of health, ministry of education, and major international donors if the country depends on donors for a significant proportion of total public revenue. The stakeholders with medium power often include the professional associations, unions and directors of hospitals and clinics. Stakeholders with low power include local governments, nongovernmental organizations and patient organizations. These power relationships will, however, differ from country to country and they will change over time.

It would be useful to prepare a general "political map" of the stakeholders' positions and power, to assess the feasibility of gaining sufficient support to effectively ratify and implement a proposed health workforce strategy. One method for producing such a map is described by Reich (1996).

There are many potential actors to be considered in a stakeholder analysis for human resources for health. The following list of stakeholders is a list of likely stakeholders in most countries; however, some categories of players may not be applicable to a stakeholder analysis in a particular country. As a guide to thinking about the power and position of stakeholders, here is given a general estimate of the characteristics of these stakeholders based on experience in various countries is given . This overview is only a suggestive list. It should be modified based on more informed assessments about the country concerned, since stakeholders' position and power are likely to vary greatly from country to country.

Ministry of health

Almost all health workforce matters affect the ministry of health, including hiring, dismissal, rotation, placement, job development, recruitment and personnel. By virtue of its central role as provider of services and its leadership role in the sector, the ministry of health is usually the major actor in health sector policies, although its own budget may be controlled by the ministry of finance and many health workforce rules may be determined by general public service agencies. Within the ministry of health, actors at multiple levels have interests in policy relating to human resources for health. Depending on the degree of decentralization, these may include administrators in central or federal offices, regional or district directors, those at lower levels of the system, hospital directors, as well as mayors, governors and local legislatures. Ministries of health have taken different positions on health workforce development, sometimes supporting staff reductions if they bring salary increases, and at other times resisting changes that might reduce the political power of patronage hiring.

Ministry of finance

The ministry of finance plays a powerful role in any policy involving the budget and the number and types of personnel posts. It will thus play a major role in health workforce policy if there is a change in the financing of health services or in the ministry of health's budget. The ministry of finance usually sees health as solely a consumption good and therefore is often not supportive of health workforce policies which involve increased budgetary expenditures on personnel.

Ministry of education

The ministry of education often controls the number of medical personnel who are trained and the curricula of the medical and other health personnel educational systems. The ministry of education may generally be supportive of change, especially since education is a key aspect of many solutions to problems of human resources for health (Egger et al., 2000). However, in some countries, the ministry of education and especially the leadership of the medical schools resist the expansion of physician training, fearing dilution of quality of training or a potential increase in competition among physicians. Faculties of professional schools may also resist increases in less qualified categories of health workers. The ministry of education, like the ministry of health, is powerful in terms of intangible and leadership resources, but often lacks financial and organizational resources.

Ministry of planning

The ministry of planning will be involved in the policy proposals especially if it involves calculations of overall economic growth or decisions about cancelling debt (Roberts, 2004) or any type of decentralization. The ministry of planning is likely to be supportive of health workforce policy if it can be shown to have associations with economic growth. On the other hand, the ministry of planning may not be supportive if there is evidence for failure. In Colombia, for instance, the ministry of planning was involved in health workforce reforms, but there was a lack of communication with the ministry of health (Schlette, 1998). The ministry of planning in many countries is powerful in areas of finance, organizational resources, leadership resources, and intangible (informational) resources.

Civil service agency (public service ministry)

The civil service agency is involved in any policy proposal that involves changes in the provisions of civil service laws and regulations. In most health workforce reforms, the civil service agency must work closely with the ministries of finance, education and health. Often, lack of coordination between the civil service agency and other governmental actors slows down the reform process. The civil service agency often resists any significant changes in the civil service rules governing many of the potential management reforms. It may be supportive of health workforce policy changes, if the health reforms accompany a general reform in the civil service rules and regulations. The level of power of the civil service agency will be specific to each country.

Donors and international agencies

Donors and international technical assistance agencies are often major stakeholders, especially in low income countries where donor resources make up a significant proportion of public expenditures. They typically use their financial resources, along with organizational, leadership, and intangible resources to influence government policies. Some examples of key players will be the larger donors such as the World Bank, the International Monetary Fund, WHO and other United Nations agencies (UNICEF, UNDP, Global Fund), the European Union, regional development banks and bilateral agencies (such as USAID, DFID) and major foundations such as the Gates Foundation. Donors have been increasingly interested in supporting health workforce policy reforms, especially if they are associated with economic development or their specific programme goals. The actions supported by donors differ from country to country. For example, in Cameroon, where the International Monetary Fund was involved in civil service reform, salary reductions and identification of ghost civil servants were introduced. In other countries, donors have supported salary increases. Donors are usually less supportive of simply paying for increases in salaries, although there have been some exceptions (Egger et al., 2000). DFID has started to cover significant salary increases in African countries, i.e. in Malawi.

Unions

Unions represent the workers in a certain specialty area. In health care, unions sometimes overlap with health professional associations but usually are organized across professions. The public sector workforce is often highly unionized and can play an important role in the reform process. It is important to understand and predict how unions will react to a change, in order to facilitate design and implementation of the reform. Unions are likely to be important supporters of increases in salaries and benefits but may not promote reforms designed to increase efficiency through increases in productivity. Countries with strong unions are also often better equipped to organize groups who favour or are against a certain policy. However, unions are not always well organized, especially if they are fragmented into competing groups; and in some authoritarian regimes they may be subject to repression.

Associations of health professionals

There are usually several health professional associations in a country. Generally, there are separate associations for physicians, nurses, midwives, pharmacists, dentists and paraprofessionals. These associations are often key players interested in salaries, quality of education and other human resources policies. Like the ministry of education and the medical faculties mentioned above, they may resist the expansion of training in their own fields, and of less-qualified human resources. Like unions, they may be well organized and powerful, or fragmented and weak. In some rare cases, they may be repressed by authoritarian measures.

Nongovernmental organizations

Depending on the public–private mix in the country concerned, nongovernmental organizations could play a large role in human resources for health. As nongovernmental organizations are often taking more of a role in the health system, they could become more powerful stakeholders. In terms of management reforms, some countries are contracting for management services from nongovernmental organizations. While there is often a degree of conflict between governmental and nongovernmental stakeholders, they may be important allies for some types of reforms.

Mayors and local governments

As more countries decentralize their health systems, mayors and local government leaders may take on more responsibility with health workforce reforms. In some countries, such reforms have transferred staff from central to local levels. If local governments have more control over financing and human resources decisions, they may become the key stakeholders for human resources reforms. In other systems, they may lobby for changes that strengthen local government control over salaries and other human resources policies. Local governments often resist "unfunded mandates" of national human resources policies if they impose requirements on local government budgets. The power of local governments varies, usually depending on their control of financing and on how well organized associations of local governments are for lobbying at the national level.

Media

The media can transform private troubles into public issues, create awareness among the public and political elites, and shape the boundaries and symbols of public debate (Roberts, 2004). Health workforce issues often attract media attention when health associations or unions are involved, and when physicians and other health workers go on strike. However, sustained media interest in health issues is rare and the media often resist attempts to voice the positions of reformers, preferring to report on problems and then presenting their own "balanced" interpretation of differing positions.

Patient organizations

Patient organizations are usually concerned about funding and access for patients with specific diseases. They seldom play important roles in human resources policies. However, if they are particularly effective organizations, a political strategy to get them to support reforms might be useful.

Hospitals and health clinics

Directors and managers of hospitals and health clinics are obvious stakeholders, with interests in health workforce policy because health workers and other administrative workers have jobs in their institutions. Hospitals and health clinics will be affected by policies such as increased job training, increased incentives, and increases in salaries. These policies will require more staff, both to implement the policies and to ensure that health workers are completing their regular work while taking advantage of the incentives. Managers' interests may differ from those of unions or professional associations. Depending on managers' control of their salary budgets and their own incentives for performance, they may be more interested in policies that improve efficiency and management control. Hospitals and health care clinics have some financial and organization power, and sometimes have access to policy-makers in the ministries.

Examples of stakeholder analysis of three different types of policy reform

In this section, we review three policy proposals as examples of how to assess the usual positions of key stakeholders in relation to particular policies. We assume that the country has insufficient health workforce staffing and a high out-migration of well-trained physicians and nurses . This discussion simply shows how to think about strategies. Policy and strategy changes should be carefully evaluated in the context of each country concerned.

Increasing the number of health workers

Increasing the number of specific types of health workers, such as health extension workers and health officers (who are not internationally competitive and therefore not likely to migrate), involves increasing funding to cover the costs of training and providing salaries and non-salary support. This will usually require a commitment to provide national budgetary support, and may also involve donor support at least for the initial phase. It is not unusual for the ministry of finance to put up some resistance to a reallocation of national resources to the health sector – which is often seen by economists in ministries of finance as a non-productive sector. Donors may be in favour of increased numbers of health workers but are often reluctant to provide funding for the routine and sustained costs of salaries. In addition, faculties of medicine – often in the ministry of education – and associations of physicians often oppose the training of less than fully qualified physicians (such as health officers), preferring high quality internationally certified medical training. In contrast, regional health officials, the managers of health clinics, and the leadership of training institutions for these types of health workers, may be in favour of expanding the numbers of such health workers.

Changing curricula or postgraduate requirements

Changing curricula or postgraduate residency requirements to upgrade quality or alter the profile of health workers might generate significant opposition from the educational institutions involved, such as faculties of medicine and non-professional training schools, but might be strongly supported by technical officers in donor organizations and by senior staff in the ministry of health.

Increasing salaries

Increasing salary levels and compensation packages (as has been done in Chile, Guinea-Bissau, Jamaica and the Philippines) is costly. Donors are unlikely to support paying salaries, although it has been reported that in Kyrgyzstan donors paid the salaries of staff implementing reforms and of staff running new associations of health professionals (Egger et al., 2000). Of 18 countries studied in a WHO report on human resources, 12 did increase salaries to resolve problems of staff shortages (Egger et al., 2000). Such policies are usually supported by unions, medical associations, the ministry of health staff, and hospital and clinic directors. They are often resisted, however, by the ministry of finance, donors, and local governments that have to fund the salary increases, as was the case for local governments in the Philippines.

Strategies for changing policies on human resources for health

Once a policy has been analysed, the key players identified, and their positions and powers assessed, the next step is to develop strategies to increase the number and power of supporters, and reduce the number and power of opponents.

One type of strategy is to develop specific policy advocacy packages to present arguments that show how the reform will be to the advantage of different stakeholders. For example, to overcome the resistance from other sectors, and the ministries of finance and planning, it might be useful to emphasize recent research demonstrating the importance of investments in health for overall economic development (Bloom et al., 2003).

A second strategy might be to delegitimize the opposition of the medical schools to expansion of their classes or the training of less qualified professionals by showing that this opposition may be based more on self-interest than on improving the health of the broader population. This argument could be presented in advocacy packages to specific policy-makers or even to the media.

Another strategy might be to compromise on the technically best reform policy so as to reduce opposition and increase support. Such a strategy might reduce the optimal numbers to be trained so that the budget demands would be lower. This might reduce opposition from the ministry of finance or planning. A smaller expansion of health workers, or a longer period to phase in the reform might not only reduce opposition, but also gain time to demonstrate the effectiveness of the reform and build more support. One recommendation for countries where overall support is low is to use donors to begin creating a supportive environment for health workforce policy. In many countries, donors have been effective in persuading governments to adopt policies of improving human resource capacities, as well as modernizing the state and opening the economy to foreign investment. Donors review government plans and budgets, in the usual process led by the World Bank and the International Monetary Fund, involving the development of a poverty reduction strategy paper as the basis for assigning priorities for international funding. In this process, the government agrees to performance objectives and is monitored in its performance by joint missions of donors. The consultations that take place establish the basis for continuing and new funding. Donor support is one way a country can begin to gain support for health workforce policies.

PART 3 Health Workforce Policy Development

There is no simple process for analysing country situations, setting priorities, selecting solutions and developing an appropriate sequence for investment to improve human resources for health. Many factors need to be taken into account, including the availability of reliable data, the technical and political feasibility of different types of policies, and the values of the key actors in the policy process. This section provides a set of guidelines for reviewing the current status against benchmarks, prioritizing the problem areas, selecting technically and politically feasible policy reforms, and developing a sequencing guide for the actions.

In order to develop a policy to improve the health workforce, we suggest a process comprising five steps:
- assessing current indicators of the status of the health workforce against benchmarks;
- developing criteria for prioritizing problems relating to human resources for health;
- choosing policies to improve the health workforce;
- sequencing the implementation of policies;
- developing a political strategy to increase support for policies.

Assessing the current status of the health workforce

Using the cross-cutting indicators and the indicators of financing, education and management, analysts should compare the country data to the benchmark data for countries with similar incomes and regional characteristics (when such benchmarks are available). This initial step should identify any major problems and begin to quantify the magnitude of the problems.

Cross-cutting problems
- How do densities of each category of health worker compare to benchmarks? Which categories are more under-staffed than others?
- Are there retention problems or shortages in qualified candidates for key categories?
- Are there significant regional differences in staffing, motivation and other areas?

Educational capacity problems
- Is the current education output insufficient to increase and – in the medium term – maintain densities of health workers?
- Is the pool of potential applicants for health professional education from secondary education adequate to expand the health workforce in specific categories?
- Is the distribution of educational capacity and output across geographical regions equitable in regard to human resources for health?
- Is the gender distribution of health professional education equitable?
- Is there sufficient management training?
- Are there coordination problems between the ministry of education and the ministry of health at national and regional levels?

Financial capacity problems
- Does the health sector have adequate funding?
- Is financing for human resources for health allocatively efficient?
- Is financing for human resources for health operationally efficient?
- Is funding for human resources for health equally distributed across geographical regions?
- Are salaries low and incentives inadequate?
- Is there sufficient funding for training capacities?
- Are there incentives to work in rural areas and emerging regions?

Management capacity problems
- Is there adequate information for policy and decision-making ?
- Is the division of roles and responsibilities for human resources for health across levels of the system appropriate ?
- Does the national level provide adequate policy guidance for lower administrative levels ?
- Are the health workforce adequately equipped with management skills appropriate to their level in the system ?
- Are good management techniques used at all levels of the system ?
- Are general working conditions and organizational climate adequate?
- Is the private sector adequately engaged (e.g. are relations with the private sector adequately defined; do public–private partnerships exist?)

Developing criteria for prioritizing problems relating to human resources for health

Once the assessment indicators have been analysed, it is important to establish criteria for prioritizing the problems. Country teams might consider the following criteria.

National priorities for the health workforce appropriate to health status problems

Many countries have recognized the Millennium Development Goals as identifying the highest health priorities. If this is the case, then human resources priorities might be to provide the categories of health workers that most appropriately address these health status problems – such as front-line primary care and community health workers, and general practitioners. If, however, the national priorities are to reduce mortality from chronic diseases, then other categories of health workers might be more important.

National priorities for the health workforce responsive to popular and patient satisfaction and financial security

It is also important to take into account non-health priorities, defined (WHO 2000) in *The world health report 2000* to include popular and patient satisfaction, and financial security of households. If these priorities are also considered, the criteria for prioritizing health workforce problems should also assess aspects seen by the population as most important, and aspects that reduce the financial burden on families. Taking these priorities into account might involve responding to popular demand for more specialists, or focusing on those categories of health workers who could reduce the need for high-cost care – such as health workers in prevention programmes for chronic diseases.

Current initiatives concerning the health workforce

It would be a mistake to assume that nothing is being done in a country prior to the health workforce assessment. Current initiatives reflect some basic priority setting, and those initiatives should be taken into account in the process of establishing priorities for moving forward. For instance, the government may already be developing new training programmes for front-line health workers, or it may have developed a new family medicine programme. If these initiatives address critical shortages identified in the review of indicators, they could be taken as a starting point for further development. It should be noted that initiatives might include more general developments, such as reform of the civil service, that might have an effect on the health sector.

Preliminary assessment of political feasibility of policies for human resources for health

With regard to political feasibility, making an initial assessment of the positions and power of the key stakeholders in order to identify major sources of support and of opposition should help identify whether or not the health workforce is on the political agenda. An initial calculation of the overall balance of support should assist in determining the magnitude and direction of proposed changes. If key stakeholders with sufficient power to stop some types of change are identified at an early stage, policy-makers should consider either developing political strategies to overcome that opposition or modifying proposed changes in order to neutralize the opposition by avoiding aspects that are objectionable.

Technical needs for increasing the quantity and quality of health workers

Priorities might also be set in accordance with the logistics of increasing the quantity and quality of health workers, irrespective of the categories selected.

The first requirement is that there is national level capacity in the ministry of health (and ministry of education, if appropriate) to make policy decisions based on evidence produced by the assessment. Without national decision-making authority and capacity, little is likely to be accomplished, even though some changes may be implemented through the private sector.

The second requirement is that the quality of training is adequate to provide appropriately skilled health workers in the relevant categories. Inadequately trained staff often contribute to problems rather than solving them. Poorly trained community workers, nurses and physicians undermine public confidence in the health system. Priority efforts might be directed to ensuring that educational and training capacities are of sufficient quality to assure well-trained health workers.

The third requirement is that working conditions, career paths, salary and other incentives are sufficient to attract and retain high-quality staff. This means ensuring that existing and new staff are motivated to do their jobs well and to continue working in the sector. Unless this is done, loss of trained staff through migration, a shift to the private sector, and a concentration of health workers in urban areas will result in the continuation of common problems in the area of human resources for health.

Choosing policies to improve the health workforce

It is often useful to start by identifying problems and setting priorities among them, and then to take a diagnostic journey to identify the causes of the priority problems. This diagnosis can be done using a diagnostic tree and asking "Why is there a problem? What caused that problem? What caused that cause? " and so on until geting financing, organizational, payment, regulation and behavioral causes that can be altered by policy changes (Roberts (2004).

In the case of health workforce reform, especially in low and lower middle income countries, it is likely that some policies can be chosen through a simplified process. The central reform is likely to focus on training of specific categories of health workers – those who will address the priority problems. Health workforce reforms are likely to require additional financing from the national or regional budgets and from donors. The options for education and training may include private sector education, but most likely an expansion of national public training programmes will be necessary. Problems of management will also require significant investment, to improve management information systems, and to provide training and leadership skills for managers.

At this stage it would be useful to do a risk assessment of the package of recommended activities. This assessment would review the key assumptions about political support, financial availability, current capabilities to educate and supply the increased numbers of health workers needed, and so on. There may be some assumptions (such as availability of donor funding) that, if they prove to be incorrect, might put the reform package at high risk of failure. There may be other assumptions that imply additional planning and activities to ensure that resources are available when needed. An overall assessment of both the political and technical risks should help establish priorities, and make clear to policy-makers the potential costs of failure. The package may be modified, depending on the tolerance for risk.

Sequencing the implementation of policies

There is no simple guide to the sequencing of reform strategies. The process of sequencing activities begins with priority setting. Giving priority to the training of some categories of health workers means that expansion of other categories needs to be delayed until the targets for the priority categories are fulfilled.

Two major choices on sequencing are (a) between slower incremental increases, and more rapid large scale increases in numbers of health workers; and (b) between increasing numbers of workers, and first investing in improving the health systems around existing workers.

A balance needs to be struck between, on the one hand, providing smaller numbers of new health workers or upgrading the training of existing workers, or a combination of both those approaches, and on the other hand massively increasing the number of new health workers. The strategy of hugely increasing the number of new health workers may take advantage of current donor and national priorities, but it risks being over-ambitious for existing capacity and unsustainable in the long run – leaving larger numbers of health workers without adequate salaries or without sufficient supplies to perform well in the future. A strategy of training smaller numbers of new health workers is safer since it would probably allow for higher quality training and be more sustainable in the long run. If the political and financial conditions are favourable, however, the opportunity to close the gap between current and ideal numbers of health workers might be lost by taking an approach involving the training of fewer new health workers.

A balance also needs to be struck between increasing the numbers of health workers, and improving the systems around them needed for them to be more effective. It is likely that financing increases will be necessary to address almost any shortfall in personnel, and might be necessary for early retirement policies if there are surpluses in some categories of health workers. Educational programmes will probably need to be expanded in order to train the required health workers. Management improvements will also be needed to improve working conditions and encourage the retention of staff.

It is useful to develop a work plan for the implementation of the recommended strategies. This plan, which can be drawn up using critical path analysis or similar planning tools, is probably best achieved though dialogue with national officials and donors to ensure realistic timing of activities.

Developing a political strategy to increase support for health workforce policies

The last step is to assess the political feasibility of the reform policies and readjust the proposed changes to the political reality. Using the *Policymaker* approach, the assessment team should determine the level of support for the recommended reforms and for their sequencing, paying particular attention to the position and power of key actors. Then political strategies need to be developed to ensure sufficient support and reduce opposition so that reforms are not only adopted, but also effectively implemented.

CONCLUSION

There is no universal best strategy for improving the health workforce, and there is no simple way of gaining sufficient political support for a proposed strategy. These guidelines to analytical and practical thinking about health workforce strategy and political feasibility are only as good as the data available and the analysts who make the assessments. If better information or a better understanding of the situation emerges from the exercise of applying the rapid assessment methods described here, then those outcomes should serve to inform policy-making for human resources for health.

ANNEX 1 Status of the Health Workforce

Level of human resources for health

Densities of health care workers that are "too high" or "too low" compared with health needs are commonly found worldwide. Most African countries, for instance, have less than one physician per 10 000 population, and ten African countries have fewer than 0.3 physicians per 10 000 population (World Bank, 1994b; Huddart & Picazo, 2003). Globally, 57 countries have fewer than 2.3 health workers per 10 000 population (WHO, 2006). A similar picture emerges when targets developed by individual countries are compared to the actual status of the health workforce. A 1998 survey of seven African countries reported high vacancy levels for health care posts, for instance up to 52.9% for nurses in Malawi and 72.9% for specialist physicians in Ghana (Dovlo, 1999; WHO, 2002).

While the link between level of the health workforce and health systems performance is intuitive, actual evidence linking the two is somewhat mixed. A recent study found inverse relationships between physician or nurse density and mortality measures, although previous studies had found either *positive* or no associations between similar densities and measures of mortality (Anand & Baernighausen, 2004). Two hypotheses may be offered to explain such findings. First, none of the studies appeared to have data on complementary elements to staffing level (such as distribution, or education and training). The inability to control for those factors (also theoretically expected to affect performance) may lead to the lack of consistent associations. Second, the link between the health care system and health outcomes is mixed (WHO 2003a). Thus while this guide operates under the underlying assumption that the level of health workers is an important element in health system performance, it is difficult to estimate the magnitude of its impact.

Distribution of human resources for health

Experiences from developing countries suggest that geographical, skills, gender and sectoral imbalances are all widespread, though it should be recognized that most studies concentrate on only a few health professions, namely physicians or nurses (Gupta et al., 2003).

Geographical maldistribution is prevalent in many developing countries. As many as half of the physicians in countries in Asia, Latin America and sub-Saharan Africa are concentrated in urban areas, even though 20% or less of the population resides in those areas (De Geyndt, 1995; Zurn et al., 2002; Gupta et al., 2003).

Evidence of a generalized *skills distribution* problem is not as clear. For instance, Huddart & Picazo (2003) relate that many African health care systems face an oversupply of "unskilled or lowly trained workers" but provide no supporting evidence. By contrast, other reports claim that many African health care systems suffer from a relative undersupply of community health care workers who need less training than clinically focused health workers. Huddart & Picazo (2003) estimate that about two thirds of Africa's burden of disease can be addressed by community health nurses who may cost about 30% less to train than professional, degree-level nurses.

Gender distribution problems also appear to be common and may adversely affect performance. Women continue to be relegated to lower-status occupations and proportionally fewer attain the professional or managerial posts generally occupied by men (Zurn et al., 2002). Yet there is evidence that female physicians achieve higher patient satisfaction ratings because of better physician–patient interactions (e.g. empathy, partnership building, information exchange and participatory decision-making) than their male counterparts (Verbrugge & Steiner, 1981; Hall et al., 1988; Roter et al., 1991; Kaplan et al., 1995). Performance along these dimensions of physician–patient interaction, in turn, has been shown to improve patient satisfaction and health outcomes (Barsky et al., 1980; Greenfield et al., 1985; Kaplan et al., 1989; Cooper-Patrick et al., 1999).

Finally, in terms of *sectoral distribution*, there is anecdotal evidence that some African governments cannot retain sufficient numbers of health workers in some categories in the public sector (such as pharmacists and pharmacy technicians) because these health workers have a much higher earning potential in industry (Huddart & Picazo, 2003). Additional indicators for assessing the status of human resources for health are suggested in the following table.

Table 12. Status of human resources for health (HRH): secondary indicators

Dimension	Indicator	Bench-mark	Reference	Comments	
				Indicator/benchmark	Source
• HRH performance (productivity)	Surgeries per operating room per day		*Indicator* • Hall (2001) *Benchmark:* • None		Can be assessed through international-ly-accessible databases, in-country databases and ministry of health documents
• HRH performance (quality)	Proportion of wound infec-tions after surgery		*Indicator* • Casparie (2000) *Benchmark:* • None		Can be assessed through international-ly-accessible databases, in-country databases and ministry of health documents

Cross-cutting problems concerning human resources for health

Attractiveness for graduates

Surveys of medical schools and nursing students suggest that both externally driven and intrinsic factors do motivate undergraduates to enter training in the health professions. Job-related aspects (e.g. job security, employment benefits and financial rewards) are balanced by personal interests (e.g. a focus on helping people, having a family member or friend who was a health professional, a desire for personal growth) (Kersten et al., 1991; Razali, 1996; Larsen et al., 2003). An additional indicator for assessing the attractiveness of the health professions is suggested in the table at the end of this section.

Migration

While estimates of migration from source countries are likely to be unreliable and may underestimate the outflows of health workers (Stilwell et al., 2003), estimates from receiving countries point to considerable migration flows. For instance, 80 000 foreign nurses are estimated to be working in the United States (ILO, 1998). There is also evidence that emigration of health personnel from developing countries is likely to persist. A survey in a number of African countries, for example, revealed that between one quarter of health personnel in Uganda and almost two thirds in Ghana expressed an intent to emigrate (WHO, 2003b).

Emigration has been documented to negatively affect the level of the health workforce and health system efficiencies. In Jamaica, 80% of trained doctors and 95% of trained nurses were lost to emigration between 1978 and 1985. Almost half the graduates from the All-India Institute of Medical Science in New Delhi subsequently left the country, and fewer than 10% of doctors trained in Zambia since its independence practise there today (ILO, 1998; Couper, 2002). Similar findings have been reported elsewhere (Ghana Ministry of Health, 2000; Huddart & Picazo, 2003). The costs of such losses – while difficult to quantify – can be inferred from training statistics. For every one physician added to its workforce, for instance, Grenada trained 22 doctors (ILO, 1998). Much like premature death from HIV/AIDS, emigration entails significant efficiency losses for a health care system.

Premature death

There have been few studies to quantify the effect of premature death (from HIV/AIDS) on the health workforce. Reports from sub-Saharan Africa, however, suggest a potentially severe constraint on health care systems: Botswana and Zambia have estimated HIV/AIDS prevalences of 20%–40% among health care workers. This has the potential to impose long-term resource drains on the health care systems of affected countries (Cohen, 2002).

Multiple job holding

The evidence describing the extent of multiple job holding is stronger than the evidence relating multiple job holding to health system performance. Multiple job holding is reportedly common in developing countries, and studies have explored its determinants across several contexts (Roenen et al., 1997; Gruen et al., 2002; Berman & Cuizon, 2004). The link between multiple job holding and its negative or positive consequences, however, rests mainly on case studies and anecdotal evidence.[1] While multiple job holding may therefore be a source of concern, it is difficult to know a priori whether it will affect the health system.

Absenteeism and ghost workers

High rates of absenteeism have been reported in various contexts across developing countries, but systematic data collection is generally lacking. Bangladesh provides an example for which health workforce absenteeism is a major problem and data are available (Begum & Sen, 1997)

Based on a national sample of unannounced visits, Chaudhury & Hammer (2003) found that physicians were absent over 40% of the time that they should have been available for service. Determinants of absenteeism in Bangladesh included accountability factors (i.e. whether a physician lived in the same village in which he or she worked) and work conditions (i.e. presence of a road and electricity). More generally, however, it is difficult to speculate on the extent of or reasons for absenteeism, as countries often do not take steps to quantify the extent of absenteeism on a nationally representative scale (Chaudhury & Hammer, 2003). Similarly, there is evidence from a few countries that ghost workers constitute a large problem. Over a quarter of the payroll in Guinea-Bissau (700 persons) were identified as ghost workers, and several other African countries are thought to have ghost workers in their health sector (Egger, 2000; World Bank, 1994b).

Motivation

Health worker motivation is viewed as a widespread problem in the public sector and in developing countries. To date, however, only a handful of studies could be located attempting to measure motivation, and none studied either its scope or its consequences for the performance of the health workforce (Franco et al., 2004).

Table 13. Cross-cutting problems concerning human resources for health (HRH): secondary indicators

Dimension	Indicator	Bench-mark	Reference	Comments	
				Indicator/ benchmark	Source
• Attractiveness of profession	Mean applicant grade point average	None currently available		Categories include, but are not limited to: physicians, nurses, midwives, health assistants, front-line workers, physician specialists, pharmacists	Can be assessed through internationally-accessible databases, in-country databases and ministry of health documents, or by panel of experts or other methods of estimation

---

[1] Potential positive consequences of multiple job holding include increased use of health services through the use of the private sector services, continued provision of governmental services at below-market prices (but with the same personnel as private sector facilities), and the chance for providers to gain experience or skills through private sector practice (Berman & Cuizon, 2004).

ANNEX 2 Financial policy levers affecting the Health Workforce

Salary level as a determinant of the level of health workers

The level of health workers available in a country is most appropriately measured by the total number of hours available for health work in a given time period (e.g. a week). The total number of hours available is determined by the number of health workers as well as by the number of hours any one health worker spends per time period working in his or her profession (work intensity):

> number of hours of health work per period = number of health workers × number of hours worked per health worker.

The number of health workers is determined by several of the factors described earlier. Decreasing the attractiveness of the health professions decreases the number of entrants into the health workforce. Net out-migration reduces the number of health workers, as do early retirement and job changes. Absenteeism,[1] on the other hand, will reduce the number of hours worked per health worker. All these cross-cutting factors are likely to be influenced by the salary level as well as relevant non-salary expenditures in a particular country.

Overall, most individual studies that provide evidence about the link between salary level and a specific exit, entry or intensity factor are observational, and their conclusions are limited to a certain time, geographic location and category of health workers. Thus, the evidence cited below identifies possible causal links, but should not be generalized to other contexts without further investigation. Some additional indicators are suggested in the table at the end of the annex.

Migration

Salary differentials between recipient and source country are among the most commonly identified and important reasons for migration. High salaries in a recipient country are a pull-factor for migration (Buchan et al., 2003).

In surveys in six African countries (Cameroon, Ghana, Senegal, South Africa, Uganda and Zimbabwe), salary level is the most commonly given reason for intention to migrate (between 68% and 84% of respondents) (WHO, 2003b). PAHO (2001) found that poor pay was among the most important push factors for migration from the Caribbean. Similarly, Buchan et al. (2003) report that, in focus groups held in Norway and Ireland with nurses from the Philippines, the ability to earn higher salaries was given as the main factor motivating migration.

Job satisfaction, job change and early retirement

A large number of studies suggest that salary levels are among the most important determinants of job satisfaction among a number of health workers in a variety of contexts, including government physicians in Malaysia (Sararaks & Jamaluddin, 1999), nurses in the United Kingdom (Callaghan, 2003), home health nurses in the United States (Juhl et al., 1993), school nurses (Junious et al., 2004) and rural public health nurses in China (Lee et al., 1991). Similarly, salary levels have been found to be a principal reason for dissatisfaction among registered nurses in Lebanon (Yaktin et al., 2003), school nurses (Munro, 1983), nurse practitioners in the United States (Tri, 1991), and physicians, nurses, pharmacists, and medical laboratory technologists in Kuwait (Shah et al., 2001).

---

[1] Multiple job holding will decrease the number of hours per health worker only if second jobs are not in health care. If second jobs are in health care, as in the case of simultaneous job holdings in the private and public sectors, they may increase the number of hours worked per health worker.

There is some evidence that dissatisfaction with low salaries may lead to job change or early retirement. For instance, based on interviews with nurses in three London hospitals, Mackereth (1989) concludes that low salary levels and working conditions are the most important reasons for considering leaving the nursing profession. Parker & Rickman (1995) find that the following factors have a significant influence on the probability of withdrawal of registered nurses from the workforce in the United States: salary rate, other family income, presence of children, and full-time or part-time work status. Following in-depth interviews with nurses, Cangelosi et al. (1998) conclude that low salaries and poor staffing are the two most important factors motivating nurses to leave their jobs. Similarly, a study among dental hygiene workers in Texas concludes that low salary levels and lack of benefits are among the factors motivating workers to leave dental hygiene practice for another job (Johns et al., 2001).

A few studies have produced nuanced results. For instance, a survey among front-line public health nurses in rural British Columbia suggests that while low salary levels are the main reason for job dissatisfaction, this dissatisfaction does not lead the nurses to quit their jobs unless they have additional economic or family reasons to do so (Henderson Betkus & MacLeod, 2004). Another study among nurses in rural areas of the United States concludes that autonomy (and not salary level) is the most effective predictor of intention to remain in the current position (Hanson et al., 1990).

In sum, salary levels (absolute or relative) are likely to be an important predictor of retention of health workers. However, in a particular context among a particular group of health workers, this may not be true.

Attractiveness of the health professions

The link between the attractiveness of the health professions and salary levels seems plausible, but has not been studied extensively. One survey among United States high school seniors found that salary level and dislike of being close to dying people were the main reasons for seniors not to choose nursing as a future profession (Stevens & Walker, 1993).

Salary level as a determinant of the distribution of health workers

Geographical distribution

There is some evidence about a causal link between salaries (and other financial incentives) and the geographical distribution of the health workforce. Lower salaries in rural areas have been found to be an important factor discouraging rural practice. For instance, Siziya & Woelk (1995) in a study of medical students and junior doctors in Zimbabwe find that three factors make working in rural areas unattractive to the health workers interviewed: lower salaries, lower standard of living, and the lower prestige of rural as opposed to urban practice. In another study in Zimbabwe, Mutziwa-Mangiza (1998) finds that many Zimbabwean junior and middle-level doctors who would normally not choose to work in rural hospitals in South Africa, do so solely because of the higher financial rewards.

Salary differentials between rural and urban areas have also been successfully used as a policy lever to reduce geographical imbalances in the distribution of the health workforce. For instance, in Indonesia a bonus of up to 100% of the normal salary attracted medical graduates from Jakarta to the outer islands (Chomitz, 1998). Findings by Gruen et al. (2002) suggest that financial incentives would be successful among recent graduates as a motivator to practise in rural areas. In the United States, Jackson et al. (2003) report that financial incentives have been successful in motivating physicians to practise in underserved rural areas in West Virginia.

On the one hand, financial incentives may be an appropriate lever to use in order to motivate health workers to practise in rural settings, because they signal the social value of service and provide a sense of recognition (Adams & Hicks, 2000). On the other hand, while financial incentives may be successful, they may have a number of disadvantages. First, they are expensive; the higher rural salaries need to compensate health workers not only for the perceived reduced quality of life and reduced potential for professional development, but also for the loss of additional sources of income, which are available in the cities but are lacking in the countryside (Roenen et al., 1997). Second, financial incentives may attract health workers to rural areas who are inappropriately skilled or motivated (Chomitz, 1998). Evidence exists that long-term rural retention may be less influenced by salary levels and more by educational and demographic factors, such as medical school curricula or rural background (Humphreys et al. 2001; Brooks et al. 2002). See also Annex 3.

Skill distribution

Without listing sources or providing specific country examples, Huddart & Picazo (2003) claim that one problem facing a number of African health care systems is an oversupply of "unskilled or lowly trained workers" who are relatively well paid in comparison to their highly trained colleagues. This salary compression constitutes an obstacle to pay increases in the public health sector. By contrast, other reports claim that many African health care systems suffer from a relative undersupply of front-line health care workers, who need less training than clinically focused health workers. Huddart & Picazo (2003) estimate that about two thirds of Africa's burden of disease could be addressed by community health nurses, who may cost about 30% less to train than professional, degree-level nurses.

Evidence on the substitution of health workers of different skill levels – in respect of health care costs and outcomes – exists mainly with regard to the substitution of unlicensed nurse assistants for registered nurses, and the substitution of clinical nurses and physician assistants for general practitioners. Overall, the evidence is mixed. Moreover, most of the studies have been undertaken in developed countries (Buchan & Dal Poz, 2002).

Nurse aides have been found to achieve cost savings and not to adversely affect patient satisfaction (Hesterly & Robinson, 1990; Bostrom & Zimmerman 1993). By contrast, other studies report that highly qualified nurses are associated with higher quality of care (Carr-Hill et al., 1995). Three recent randomized controlled trials which compared nurse practitioners with general practitioners found that overall, nurse practitioners achieved quality of care comparable to general practitioners, but were less costly per time unit, or achieved higher patient satisfaction because they spent more time per patient (Kinnersley et al. 2000; Shum et al., 2000; Venning et al. 2000).

There is evidence that salary differentials between different categories of health workers may cause imbalances in distribution. For instance, in the United States, where a number of specialty physicians earn about twice as much as family physicians, residency programmes have been increasingly unable to fill positions for training in family medicine. The declining interest of graduates of United States medical schools in family medicine residencies has been largely attributed to the lower salaries family physicians earn relative to their colleagues in other specialties (Pugno & McPherson, 2002).

Gender distribution

Salary levels may play an important role in the gender distribution of the health workforce. In a review of the studies that look into reasons why fewer men than women choose nursing as a profession, Villeneuve (1994) shows that salary levels are a main deterrent for men to become nurses. However, the study also shows that salary levels may be an equally important concern for women in considering a nursing career. The cultural understanding of nursing as a female profession may be a more important factor determining the gender imbalance in nursing.

A number of studies have demonstrated that there are significant differences in salary levels between men and women working in health sector jobs, given like responsibilities. For instance women with a Master of Public Health or a Master of Health Administration earn less then their male colleagues in their first job, after differences in human capital have been taken into account. This salary differential seems to persist or to widen as the years since graduation increase (Bradley et al., 2000). The different salary levels of female and male health workers may be one factor determining a lower proportion of women in some health professions. However, evidence as to whether this is really the case is lacking.

Sectoral distribution

It seems likely that a salary differential between the public and private sectors will lead to more vacancies in the less well-paying sector. For instance, a nurse in Zimbabwe in 1998 could expect to earn 40% more in the private as opposed to the public sector. There is anecdotal evidence that some African governments cannot retain sufficient numbers of health workers in some categories in the public sector (such as pharmacists and pharmacy technicians) because these workers have a much higher earning potential in industry (Huddart & Picazo, 2003).

Salary level as a determinant of the performance of health workers

In terms of performance, salary levels may have a direct and positive impact as well as an indirect and negative impact on the efficiency of the health workforce. On the one hand, increased salaries may increase efficiency because they raise motivation and reduce such coping mechanisms as multiple job holding. On the other hand, financial efficiency (i.e. the hours done by health workers per money spent) will, other things being equal, decrease as the salary level increases. Some additional indicators are suggested in the table at the end of the annex.

Multiple job holding

Salary levels have been found to have an important influence on decisions by health workers to simultaneously hold multiple jobs, e.g. in both the public and private sectors. One common strategy physicians use to cope with underpayment in the public sector is to moonlight in the private sector (Ferrinho et al., 1998; Van Lerberghe et al., 2002b). Moonlighting in the private sector has become prevalent in a number of health care systems which underwent a rapid liberalization of medical practice, such as those in Malawi, Mozambique and the United Republic of Tanzania (Huddart & Picazo, 2003). Roenen et al. (1997) identify 28 different strategies which doctors from different countries in Sub-Saharan Africa employ to generate income in addition to their relatively low public salary. These including multiple job holding, private practice, allowances, per diems, and gifts from patients. Roenen and colleagues report that the majority of these strategies enable doctors to earn incomes that are much higher than their public sector salaries. At the same time, many of the strategies divert resources (time and materials) from the public sector to the private sector and thus lower the efficiency of public sector provision.

Raising salary levels could theoretically be successful as a means of reducing multiple job holding. In a survey of doctors who hold jobs in the public as well as in the private sector in Bangladesh, Gruen et al. (2002) find that primary care physicians would probably give up private practice and concentrate on work in the public sector if their salaries in the public sector increased. Secondary and tertiary health care workers appear to be less likely to give up private practice in response to a public sector salary increase.

Motivation

Low motivation of health workers to work hard and well may be an important obstacle to efficiency in a health care system. Motivation is a complex mechanism which may be influenced by a range of financial and non-financial incentives. The salary level may serve as one factor (albeit a very crude one) influencing motivation. For instance, a study in Viet Nam (Dieleman et al., 2003) found that the most important factors which motivate health workers in rural areas include appreciation by others, job stability, income, and training. Low salaries and difficult working conditions were found to be factors discouraging good work performance. In a similar vein, salaries which are perceived to be unfair (either in absolute terms or in comparison to other locations or other occupations) may result in poor motivation. For example, in a study in South Africa, Bachmann & Makan (1997) found that perceived salary inequalities across different health organizations diminish the potential for cooperation between different health organizations, which would result in efficiency gains.

Informal payments

Low level of public sector pay has been implicated as increasing the prevalence of informal payments (Colclough, 1997). There is evidence that one main reason for accepting (or asking for) informal payments in China is to compensate for pay perceived as low (Zhou & Zhang, 1994).

Absenteeism

Although it may seem plausible that low salary levels may increase the probability of absenteeism, there is no evidence that this is in fact the case.

Ghost workers

There is evidence from a few countries that ghost workers (individuals who receive salaries but do not exist as real health workers) constitute a large problem. A study in Guinea-Bissau identified 700 ghost workers, constituting over a quarter of the payroll (Egger et al., 2000). The World Bank (1994b) listed a number of African countries as having ghost workers in their health sector: Cameroon, the Central African Republic, the Gambia, Ghana, Senegal and Uganda.

Non-salary expenditures

Emigration has been found to be determined by continuing education opportunities, working environment, health sector resources and workload, in addition to salary levels (WHO, 2003b). Other factors motivating emigration include improved pensions, child care, and recognition (Bundred & Levitt, 2000; Van Lerberghe et al., 2002b; Stilwell et al., 2003). Recent evidence from Ghana and South Africa suggests that the fear of contracting HIV in high HIV-prevalence countries as well as the fear of contracting other bloodborne viruses (hepatitis B and C) may be an important dimension of dissatisfaction with workplace conditions, factoring into migration decisions (Stilwell et al., 2003; Vujicic et al., 2004).

In addition to the indirect effect of HIV/AIDS on health workforce levels through its influence on migration and entry into the profession, the pandemic directly affects the level of human resources for health. For instance, in Malawi 45% of health worker deaths have been reported to be attributable to HIV/AIDS (Malawi Ministry of Health and Population, and Department of Planning, 2001). A study in Zambia found that the risk of HIV-infection among surgeons is 15% higher than in developed countries (Consten et al., 1995). It has been estimated that African health systems may lose 20% of their health workforce to HIV/AIDS in the coming years (Tawfik & Kinoti, 2003; Joint Learning Initiative, 2004).

Another case in point is the distribution of health workers. The case of Thailand suggests that a combination of measures may successfully improve the rural–urban maldistribution. Many of these measures will lead to non-salary health sector expenditures, e.g. training opportunities and improved health infrastructure (Joint Learning Initiative, 2004).

As these examples demonstrate, a number of the non-salary determinants of health workforce level, distribution and performance can be addressed within the health care sector (see also Annexes 3 and 4).

Table 14. Financing of human resources for health (HRH): secondary indicators

Dimension	Indicator	Bench-mark	Reference	Comments	
				Indicator/ benchmark	Source
• Migration: salary level	• % of health workers intending to emigrate who list salary level as a main reason • % of health workers who are emigrant nationals listing salary level as a main reason	None	None	Benchmark types: • cross-profession • time series Additional information: • salary level which interviewees feel would be sufficient for them not to migrate • other changes which interviewees feel could prevent them from migrating	Special studies, scientific publications

Dimension	Indicator	Bench-mark	Reference	Comments	
				Indicator/ benchmark	Source
• Job change and early retirement: salary level	• % of health workers intending to change jobs or retire early who list salary level or benefits as main motivators	None	None	Benchmark types: • cross-profession Additional information: • salary level which would be sufficient to convince interviewees not to change jobs or retire early • other changes which could convince interviewees not to change jobs or retire early	Special studies, scientific publications
• HRH efficiency: skill distribution	• Proportion of different skill levels of HRH	None	None	Benchmark types: • cross-country • current evidence	Can be assessed through internationally-accessible databases, in-country databases and ministry of health documents
• Skill distribution: salary level	• Relative average salary level of different skill-levels of HRH	None	None	Benchmark types: • cross-country Additional information: • reasons given for choosing or not choosing certain skill levels	Can be assessed through internationally-accessible databases, in-country databases and ministry of health documents
• Sector distribution: salary level	• Ratio of average public:private salary levels by HRH category	None	None	Additional information: • reasons given for choosing or not choosing certain skill levels	Can be assessed through internationally-accessible databases, in-country databases and ministry of health documents
• Multiple job holding: salary level	• Ratio of average public: private non-salary benefits by HRH category • % HRH stating that they hold more than one job	None	None	Additional information: • willingness to quit additional jobs, if salary level in first job were high enough • salary level needed to prevent multiple job holding • other factors causing multiple job holding	Can be assessed through internationally-accessible databases, in-country databases and ministry of health documents, special studies, scientific publications
• Ghost workers	• Ghost worker density (from a comparison of a staffing inventory with the payroll)	None	None	Benchmark types: • cross-country • political target	Can be assessed through in-country databases and ministry of health documents, special studies, scientific publications

ANNEX 3 | Educational policy levers affecting the Health Workforce

Pool of potential applicants

The pool of potential applicants for different educational tracks leading to different careers in health is defined as those students graduating in one year who would theoretically be eligible to attend a specific training institution, such as a medical school (number of graduating high school students), a nursing school (number of graduating middle school students), or a residency programme (number of graduating medical school students). In addition, the pool includes:

- people who after a first non-health care career decide to enter a career in health care;
- people who intend to switch from one health care job to another;
- people who are currently training for a job that is not in health care, but intend to switch to a health care job.

The pool of potential applicants itself is likely to be a constraint. Health education decision-makers may not be able to influence a country's student intake to secondary education.

Application rate

The application rate is the proportion of applicants to a health educational institution out of the total pool of potential applicants. One important cause of low application rates may be the high cost of education for a job in health care relative to the cost of education for another occupation, or to the income that could be earned by directly entering the workforce.

Both the attractiveness of the health professions and obstacles to receiving a health-related education have been found to affect the decisions of prospective entrants. In countries where medical education is free, for example, the cost of books and other learning tools can still be substantial, as can the opportunity costs of deferring entry to the workforce (Wahba, 2003).

There is also some observational evidence that the application rate for a certain specialization can be increased by the selection of the content of a medical education programme. For instance, the problem-based and community-oriented innovations in the medical curriculum at the University of New Mexico in the United States are reported to have increased application rates for careers in primary care, rural medicine and work with underserved populations (Kaufman et al., 1989).

Institutional acceptance rate

The institutional acceptance rate is the proportion of applicants who are accepted into the health education institution to which they applied. This rate will be bounded by the maximum number of places which can be offered to applicants, as well as by the quality of the applicants. Applicant quality, in turn, depends upon the quality of students who have completed secondary schools and the attractiveness of the health profession.

There is some evidence from southern African countries that the number of medical school places and the number of medical educators has been reduced in the recent past in order to cut government spending, and that this reduction is now jeopardizing the ability of these countries to accept the number of medical students that would be needed to meet national needs for health workers (Padarath et al., 2003).

Student acceptance rate

The student acceptance rate is the proportion of students who start their education in a programme into which they have been accepted. The nationwide student acceptance rate can differ from the institution acceptance rate for two reasons: graduates may have been accepted into more than one educational programme or graduates may decide not to pursue health-related education despite a successful application.[1] Prospective students who, despite a successful application, do not pursue education in the field of health may be deterred by the unattractiveness of the profession.

Success rate

The success rate is the proportion of entrants into a certain health education programme who finish the programme successfully. It equals one minus the sum of the drop-out rates in each of the years from the start to the end of the health education programme. The success rate (or the drop-out rate) will be determined by characteristics of the health education programme as well as by the motivation and abilities of the students. One important reason for drop-out is a focus on theoretical knowledge while neglecting practical skills. Students may feel discouraged by the apparent disconnect between their education and the skills they will need in the workforce, and may decide to leave the programme (Majoor, 2004).

There is evidence that student-centred and skill-centred educational programmes have lower median study times and lower drop-out rates than more traditional educational programmes (Dolmans & Schmidt, 1996; Kruseman et al., 1997). Future work conditions, social status and income may also play an important role in determining the drop-out rate. It is estimated that the attrition rate during medical education in the United States is 1.1%, while it is around 30% in Ethiopia (Barzansky et al., 1999; Wahba, 2003).

Entry rate

The entry rate equals the proportion of graduates who enter the workforce of the health profession for which they were trained. It consists of a national entry rate (i.e. the proportion of graduates who work in their field of training in the country in which they trained) and an international entry rate (i.e. the proportion of graduates who work in their field of training but not in the country in which they trained). The national entry rate will depend upon the perception of recent graduates of working in the health field. Possible determinants of entry include perceived workload, professional respect during residency and the attractiveness of a health career compared to feasible alternatives.

There is evidence that bureaucratic regulations may discourage young graduates from entering or continuing medical practice in their country of training (Ndumbe, 2003). The international entry rate (and migration), in contrast, will depend on the attractiveness of working in the health field nationally relative to working in the health field in another country. The educational system can prevent migration to some extent by training health workers specifically for national health care needs (while explicitly not focusing on technical skills and knowledge of diseases which do not add much to the national burden of disease) (Majoor, 2004).

Quality of graduates (knowledge and skills)

A number of frameworks have been proposed to assess the quality of health care education. Among them, we chose the WFME standards (WFME, 2001) as a starting point for identifying indicators of the quality of health care education (see main text for reasons). There is an incomplete overlap between the WFME's nine areas of quality of education and the areas proposed in other documents (listed below). Therefore we have selectively incorporated suggestions from other documents.

---

[1] If all applicants applied to only one educational programme and started that programme (conditional upon acceptance), the student acceptance rate would equal the institutional acceptance rate.

Source	Areas of assessment of educational quality
Accreditation Council for Graduate Medical Education (2004)	• Patient care • Medical knowledge • Practice-based learning and improvement • Interpersonal and communication skills • Professionalism • System-based practice
Harris (1978)	• Purposes and objectives • Governance • Validity of degrees • Adequate resources • Stability • Integrity
Lawrence & Green (1980)	• Scholarly productivity of academic staff • Other achievements of academic staff • Institutional resources • Programme efficiency • Outcomes
Troutt (1979)	• Purposes and objectives • Educational programme • Financial resources • Academic staff • Library or learning resources

Council of Graduate Schools in the United States (1977)	• Quality of academic staff
	• Facilities
	  –Library and computer
	  –Physical
	  –Auxiliary
	• Doctoral programme
	  –Courses
	  –Admissions
	  –Residency
	  –Examinations
	  –Dissertations

Frank (2005)	• Academic staff • Students • Academic programme • Resources

The following table provides additional indicators that may be used to assess quality of education.

Table 15. Education of human resources for health (HRH): secondary indicators of quality of education

Dimension	Indicator	Bench-mark	Reference	Comments	
				Indicator/ benchmark	Source
• HRH distribution: gender distribution	Proportion of females enrolled in secondary school (gross)	50% (equality) 42% (average of low income countries) 46% (average of middle income countries) 49% (average of high income countries)	*Bench-mark:* • World Bank (2004)	Informs about a potential root cause of inequality in gender distribution of HRH	Can be assessed through ministry of education documents, HRH education institution documents or interviews with HRH school administrators
• HRH performance: Mission and objectives (academic autonomy)	Policy of academic autonomy	Existence	*Indicator:* • WFME (2003) (adapted)	The academic staff of the medical school should have academic freedom, within the boundaries set by the mission statement and objectives, to design the curriculum and allocate resources for its implementation	Can be assessed through document review or key informant interviews at HRH education institutions
• HRH performance: Educational programme (instructional methods)	Student responsibility for learning	None	*Indicator:* • WFME (2003) (adapted)	The instructional methods should train students to take responsibility for their learning progress	Can be assessed through document review or key informant interviews at HRH education institutions or observation of teaching sessions
• HRH performance: Educational programme (clinical sciences and skills)	Health promotion, prevention, public health, and alternative medical practice	Existence	*Indicator:* • WFME (2003) (adapted)	Some components of the clinical sciences curriculum should be concerned with health promotion, prevention, public health, and alternative medical practice	Can be assessed through document review or key informant interviews at HRH education institutions
• HRH performance: Educational programme (clinical sciences and skills)	Integration of basic sciences and clinical sciences	Existence	*Indicator:* • WFME (2003) (adapted)	Basic science teaching should focus on clinically relevant topics, and clinical science teaching should include links to the basic sciences	Can be assessed through document review or key informant interviews at HRH education institutions

Dimension	Indicator	Bench-mark	Reference	Comments	
				Indicator/ benchmark	Source
• HRH per-formance: Educational programme (continuing education)	Participa-tion rate in continuing education programmes, by HRH category	None	None	Cross-country	Can be assessed through national and sub-national physi-cian organizations
• HRH per-formance: Educational programme (clinical sciences and skills)	Coaching and mentor-ing schemes	Existence			Can be assessed through document re-view or key informant interviews at HRH education institutions
• HRH per-formance: Educational resources (research)	Opportu-nities for students to participate in research	Existence			Can be assessed through document re-view or key informant interviews at HRH education institutions
• HRH per-formance: Educational resources (educational exchanges)	Links with other HRH education institutions	Number of national links, number of interna-tional links	*Indicator:* • WFME (2003) (adapted)	The HRH education institu-tion should have exchange programmes and other collaborations with other national and international HRH education institutions	Can be assessed through document re-view or key informant interviews at HRH education institutions
• HRH per-formance: Educational resources (physical facilities)	Student and staff feedback on facilities	Existence	*Indicator:* • WFME (2003) (adapted)		Can be assessed through document re-view or key informant interviews at HRH education institutions
• HRH per-formance: Educational resources (review)	Mechanism to review ba-sic sciences and clinical sciences resources	Existence	*Indicator:* • WFME (2003) (adapted)		Can be assessed through document re-view or key informant interviews at HRH education institutions

ANNEX 4 Management policy levers affecting the Health Workforce

Public sector context

The impact of civil service reforms – especially decentralization – on human resources reveals a complicated picture. On the one hand, decentralization may inhibit system performance. Commonly, concerns cited by affected staff revolve around system insufficiencies (e.g. salaries, staff, equipment), heightened inequities, favouritism or perceived fairness, and loss of career control (e.g. limited authority to recruit and dismiss staff, lack of in-service training opportunities). On the other hand, if local managers do not have the power to take disciplinary actions against their personnel, for instance, there may be few incentives for staff to perform well (Martineau & Martinez, 1997). Indeed, some research indicates that managers with higher decision-making power to make staff appointments are also better performers (Diaz-Monsalve, 2003). Poor management may result if local managers gain new responsibilities without the necessary training, such as in health management information systems (Kolehmainen-Aitken, 1992, 2004; Gladwin et al., 2002).

High-level leadership in human resources management

Though few analyses of human resources management exist at the system level, there is some evidence at the institutional level that a commitment to good management is associated with positive organizational outcomes. Most notably, a series of studies on "magnet hospitals" in the United States indicates that "magnetism" (i.e. attractiveness to staff and patients) does appear to be related to better results in terms of staffing indicators, which in turn may emanate from sustained implementation of certain human resources management interventions, such as those which support nurse autonomy and encourage participatory decision-making. In other studies on nursing homes in Canada and the United States, better-performing institutions were more likely to have implemented progressive or "high performance" human resources management policies (Buchan, 2004).

Management training has also been linked to health worker performance, but the evidence base is not deeply developed. Studies from Latin American and the Caribbean suggest that management training is associated with better staff performance (measured in terms of knowledge and use of management practices), depends on how the training is implemented (e.g. pedagogical training methods used and length of training), and may be most successful when support from the central level is forthcoming (Diaz-Monsalve, 2004). Findings from China also indicate that administrative or environmental factors can limit the effects of management training on performance (Yaping & Stanton, 2002).

Core administration of human resources management

While conventional wisdom and anecdotal evidence suggests that administrative elements of human resources management are important, few studies in international health have isolated the effects of each. Nevertheless, the available evidence sheds insights into how these administrative elements might be linked to performance. Quantitative analyses have provided some evidence that clear job descriptions (alongside performance review) are linked with better performance of health sector personnel such as district health managers and maternal health care providers (Diaz-Monsalve, 2003; Fort & Voltero 2004). Career paths have been linked to personnel retention in some qualitative studies. For instance, while an adequate salary is usually the most important determinant of migration, findings from several countries indicate that a better working environment and career path are commonly cited by health workers as factors that would induce them to remain in the country (Zurn et al., 2002; Alkire & Chen, 2004; Vujicic et al., 2004). Indeed, clear-cut "merit-based career structures offering attractive posts in clinical or research fields, accompanied by adequate remuneration" have been proposed as a potential remedy to health worker migration (Marchal & Kegels, 2003).

In terms of health management information systems, significant obstacles to data collection and analysis are the norm in developing countries, which limits the potential positive impact of data management for health systems planning and operations (Sandiford et al., 1992; Azubuike & Ehiri, 1999). Inefficient or lack of use of health management information systems may indicate underlying managerial deficiencies in using data for decisions, including: irrelevance of information collected; poor use of information gathered; poor data quality; parallel information systems; and lack of timely reporting or feedback (Lippeveld et al., 2000). Indeed, improvement of a health management information system has been used as an "entry point for the improvement of managerial capabilities" in the Papua New Guinea health system (Newbrander & Thomason, 1988).

Institutional environment and institutional relations

Working conditions

High workloads have been linked to higher levels of stress, and malfunctioning or lack of supplies and equipment have been linked to decreased quality of care in both the primary health care and hospital settings (Bitera et al., 2002; Boonstra et al., 2003; English et al., 2004). Conversely, experience from the private sector indicates that good logistics management increases efficiencies and performance (Raja et al., 2000). Poor management, inadequate use of health information systems and low quality of services have been identified as causes of deficient referral systems (Ohara et al., 1998; Siddiqi et al., 2001). Research from high income countries suggests that providing information about reasons for referral, risks, and what patients can expect are important in reducing patient anxiety and increasing referral compliance, and hence the effectiveness of the referral system (Bossyns & Van Lerberghe, 2004).

Regarding indicators, this guide focuses on the referral system as a proxy for intra-group or institutional communication. While there is no universally applicable benchmark for optimal referral rates, evidence suggests that interventions with higher rates of referral exhibit significantly higher levels of communication. Patients receiving care as part of the integrated management of childhood illness in several sub-Saharan African countries were referred at rates substantially higher than the country average (Font et al., 2002). The upper end of those rates – 15% of all patients – can therefore be taken as a benchmark of more appropriate referral rates for priority interventions.

Staff rotation and turnover

While staff circulation as such may not be indicative of health workforce problems, inordinately high or low levels of circulation may have an adverse effect on system efficiency. Depending on the circumstances, rotation of staff can be both beneficial and detrimental to the performance of the health workforce. Regular staff rotation may generate positive effects, including the displacement of poor performers, introduction new knowledge and technology, and dealing with institutional entrenchment. However, extreme levels of rotation – either excessively high or low rates – among certain categories of health professionals may lead to negative consequences. These negative effects include an inability to carry out management change (because of either excessive rotation or as a result of entrenchment), higher costs of recruiting and training new staff, disruption of social and communication structures, productivity losses, and decreased satisfaction among "stayers" (Koh & Goh, 1995; Collins et al., 2000). The topic of staff rotation and turnover is not well-researched in the health sector, rendering estimates of its costs difficult to make (see Annex 1 for further discussion on the evidence base).

No studies could be found relating staff turnover to health systems performance in the context of developing countries. Evidence from developed nations is sparse and somewhat inconclusive. One study found that costs associated with staff turnover were more than 5% of a hospital's operating budget, but another study did not find any relationship between staff turnover and reduction of patient services or poor staff morale (Gray et al., 1996; Waldman et al., 2004). Nevertheless, even the latter study acknowledged the difficulties in estimating the true costs of turnover.

Organizational culture and leadership

The evidence linking organizational culture and leadership to personnel performance in the health field is mixed for two reasons. First, the differing method and concept of both organizational culture (including leadership) and performance render comparisons difficult (Zimmerman et al., 1993; Scott et al., 2003a). Second, it is difficult to assess how far documented relationships can be generalized. For instance, while some studies have found that supportive leadership is associated with better performance, other studies using different methods have found no relationship between leadership style and performance outcomes (Hartley & Kramer, 1991; Shortell et al., 1994; Stordeur et al., 2001). Similarly, though a good fit between a given organizational culture and employees' values has been linked to various performance outcomes particularly relevant to the health workforce, such as lower rates of turnover (Vandenberghe, 1999), a recent literature review found only modest overall evidence linking organizational culture to performance – and where linkages have been found, the effects do not necessarily translate into better patient outcomes (Scott et al., 2003 b).

In terms of teamwork and participatory decision-making, studies in hospital settings in high income countries have related teamwork to higher patient satisfaction with services, better functioning of personnel, and lower rates of staff turnover (Goni, 1999; Meterko et al., 2004). Studies in primary, secondary and tertiary care settings also suggest positive relationships between team-based approaches to care and organizational performance (De Geyndt, 1995; Lin & Tavrow, 2000). Research on district management practices in developing countries similarly indicates that teamwork helps to increase job satisfaction (Diaz-Monsalve, 2003), but the methods used to reach this conclusion could not be assessed.

In terms of vision, high standards and clear expectations, leadership in hospital intensive care units in the United States which sets "high standards, clarifies expectations, encourages initiative and input, and provides necessary support resources" has been found to be more efficient and have lower personnel turnover rates than other leadership styles (Shortell et al., 1994). More generally, it is felt that consistent leadership and management strategies result in higher performance than inconsistent strategies, though the evidence linking such leadership in developing countries is less well documented (Lerberghe et al., 2000; Scott et al., 2003 b).

Table 16. Management of human resources for health (HRH): secondary indicators for human resources administration

Dimension	Indicator	Bench-mark	Reference	Comments	
				Indicator/benchmark	Source
• Performance appraisal	% staff able to identify performance appraisal guidelines (or where to access them)	100%	*Benchmark:* • 100% Ideal	Knowledge of and familiarity with performance appraisal guidelines	Ideally assessed through quantitative survey; can also be assessed through key informant interviews
• Performance appraisal	% performance appraisal reviews documented or completed per health worker	100%	*Indicator:* • Hornby & Forte (2000) *Benchmark:* • 100% ideal	Following performance appraisal guidelines is important for the performance appraisal system to function properly	Ideally assessed through quantitative survey; can also be assessed through key informant interviews or non-probabilistic study
• Career path	% staff able to identify career path for their position (or where to locate relevant documentation)	100%	*Benchmark:* • 100% ideal	Knowledge of career path is important for effective functioning of job classification system	Ideally assessed through quantitative survey; can also be assessed through key informant interviews or non-probabilistic study

Dimension	Indicator	Bench-mark	Reference	Comments	
				Indicator/ benchmark	Source
• Payroll	Number of mechanisms in place to ensure that payroll records are accurate, rational and up-to-date (e.g. employees at correct rate of pay, noting employees transferred, dismissed or retired)	None	*Indicator:* • World Bank (2003) (adapted) *Benchmark:* • None		Ideally assessed through quantitative survey; can also be assessed through key informant interviews or non-probabilistic study
• Working conditions	% difference between stock on hand and stock recorded in inventory system	0%	*Indicator:* • DELIVER/ John Snow (2002) (adapted) *Benchmark:* 0% ideal	Indicator of system-level management capacities that affect facility-level performance	Can be assessed through document review (e.g. pharmaceutical management study) or key informant interviews
• Working conditions	% facilities with acceptable storage facilities (adequate shelving, refrigeration, electricity)	100%	*Indicator:* • DELIVER/ John Snow (2002) (adapted) *Benchmark:* 100% ideal	Indicator of system-level management capacities that affect facility-level performance	Can be assessed through document review (e.g. pharmaceutical management study) or key informant interviews
• Staff rotation	Mean time at post (by job grade)	None currently available			Can be assessed through in-country databases and ministry of health documents, or by panel of experts or other methods of estimation
• Teamwork and participatory decision-making	% staff participation in staff meetings	100%	*Benchmark:* 100% ideal	Participation of both technical and non-technical staff in staff meetings is important for effective facility-level management of the health workforce	Ideally assessed through survey; can also be assessed through document review (e.g. quarterly reports) or key informant interviews

REFERENCES

Accreditation Council for Graduate Medical Education (2004). *Outcomes project.* (http://www.acgme.org/Outcome/, accessed 21 November 2005).

Adams O, Hicks V (2000). *Pay and non-pay incentives, performance and motivation.* Paper prepared for the WHO's workshop on a Global Health Workforce Strategy, Annecy, France, World Health Organization.

Alkire S, Chen L (2004). *"Medical exceptionalism" in international migration: should doctors and nurses be treated differently?* Boston, Harvard University Asia Center.

Anand S, Bärnighausen T (2004). Human resources and health outcomes: cross-country econometric study. *Lancet*, 364: 1603-09.

Anand S, Bärnighausen T (2007). Health workers and vaccination coverage in developing countries: an econometric analysis. *Lancet*; 369, pp. 1277-85

Azubuike MC, Ehiri JE (1999). Health information systems in developing countries: benefits, problems, and prospects. *Journal of the Royal Society of Health*, 119:180–184.

Bachmann MO, Makan B (1997). Salary inequality and primary care integration in South Africa. *Social Science and Medicine*, 45:723–729.

Barsky AJ et al. (1980). Evaluating the interview in primary care medicine. *Social Science and Medicine [Medical Psychology and Medical Sociology]*, 14A:653–658.

Barua A et al. (2003). Implementing reproductive and child health services in rural Maharashtra, India: a pragmatic approach. *Reproductive Health Matters*, 11:140–149.

Barzansky B et al. (1999). Educational programs in US medical schools, 1998-1999. *Journal of the American Medical Assocation*, 282:840–846.

Bass BM, Avolio BJ (1990). *Transformational leadership development: manual for the multifactor leadership questionnaire.* Palo Alto, CA, Consulting Pyschologists Press.

Begum S, Sen B (2000). *Not quite, not enough: financial allocation and the distribution of resources in the health sector.* Dhaka: Bangladesh Institute of Development Studies/World Health Organization.

Berman P, Cuizon D (2004). *Multiple public-private jobholding of health care providers in developing countries.* London, UK Department for International Development, Health Systems Resource Centre: 1–40.

Bitera R et al. (2002). Qualité de la prise en charge des maladies sexuellement transmises: enquête auprès des soignants de six pays de l'Afrique de l'Ouest (Evaluation of sexually transmitted disease management in six countries in west Africa). *Cahiers Santé*, 12:233–239.

Bloom G et al. (2003). *How health workers earn a living in China.* Sussex, Department for International Development, University of Sussex.

Bodur S (2002). Job satisfaction of health care staff employed at health centres in Turkey. *Occupational Medicine (Oxford, England)*, 52:353–355.

Boonstra E et al. (2003). Syndromic management of sexually transmitted diseases in Botswana's primary health care: quality of care aspects. *Tropical Medicine and International Health*, 8:604–614.

Bossert T (1998). Analyzing the decentralization of health systems in developing countries: decision space, innovation and performance. *Social Science and Medicine*, 47:1513–1527.

Bossert T et al. (2004). *Human resources health systems capacity assessment, recommendations and sequencing – Ethiopia.* Boston, MA, International Health Systems Program, Harvard School of Public Health.

Bossert TJ, Beauvais JC (2002). Decentralization of health systems in Ghana, Zambia, Uganda and the Philippines: a comparative analysis of decision space. *Health Policy and Planning*, 17:14–31.

Bossert TJ et al. (2003). Decentralization and equity of resource allocation: evidence from Colombia and Chile. *Bulletin of the World Health Organization*, 81(2):95-100.

Bossyns P, Van Lerberghe W (2004). The weakest link: competence and prestige as constraints to referral by isolated nurses in rural Niger. *Human Resoures for Health*, 2:1.

Bostrom, J, Zimmerman J (1993). Restructuring nursing for a competitive health care environment. *Nursing Economics*, 11:35–41, 54.

Bradley EH et al. (2000). The role of gender in MPH graduates' salaries. *Journal of Health Administration Education*, 18:375–389.

Brooks RG et al. (2002). The roles of nature and nurture in the recruitment and retention of primary care physicians in rural areas: a review of the literature. *Academic Medicine* , 77:790–798.

Buchan J (2004). What difference does ("good") HRM make? *Human Resources for Health* , 2:6.

Buchan J, Dal Poz MR (2002). Skill mix in the health care workforce: reviewing the evidence. *Bulletin of the World Health Organization*, 80:575–580.

Buchan J et al. (2003). *International nurse mobility. trends and policy implications*. Geneva, World Health Organization.

Bundred PE, Levitt C (2000). Medical migration: who are the real losers? *Lancet*, 356:245–246.

Callaghan M (2003). Nursing morale: what is it like and why? *Journal of Advanced Nursing Nursing*, 42:82–89.

Cangelosi JD Jr et al. (1998). Factors related to nurse retention and turnover: an updated study. *Health Marketing Quarterly*, 15:25–43.

Carr-Hill RA et al. (1995). The impact of nursing grade on the quality and outcome of nursing care. *Health Economics*, 4:57–72.

Casparie, AF (2000). Postoperative wound infections: a useful indicator of quality of care?, Ned Tijdschr Geneeskd., 144(10), pp. 460-2.

Chaudhury N, Hammer J (2003). *Ghost doctors: absenteeism in Bangladeshi health facilities*. Washington, DC, World Bank.

Chomitz K (1998). *What do doctors want? Developing incentives for doctors to serve in Indonesia's rural and remote areas*. Washington, DC, World Bank.

Clark KE, Clark MB (1990). *Measures of leadership*. West Orange, NJ, Leadership Library of America.

Cohen D (2002). *Human capital and the HIV epidemic in sub-Saharan Africa*. Geneva, ILO Programme on HIV/AIDS and the World of Work.

Colclough C (1997). *Public-sector pay and adjustment: lessons from five countries*. London, New York, Routledge.

Collins CD et al. (2000). Staff transfer and management in the government health sector in Balochistan, Pakistan: problems and context. *Public Administration and Development*, 20:207–220.

Consten EC et al. (1995). A prospective study on the risk of exposure to HIV during surgery in Zambia. AIDS, 9:585–588.

Cooper RA (2003). Impact of trends in primary, secondary, and postsecondary education on applications to medical school. II: considerations of race, ethnicity, and income. *Academic Medicine*, 78:864–876.

Cooper-Patrick L et al. (1999). Race, gender, and partnership in the patient-physician relationship.Journal of the American Medical Association , 282:583–589.

Council of Graduate Schools in the United States (1977). *The doctor of philosophy degree*. Washington, DC, Council of Graduate Schools in the United States.

Couper I (2002). *The ethics of international recruitment. Paper prepared for the ARRWAG Conference in Adelaide, Australia*. South Africa, Department of Family Medicine and Primary Health Care, Medical University of Southern Africa.

De Geyndt W (1995). *Managing the quality of health care in developing countries*. Washington, DC, World Bank.

DELIVER/John Snow International (2002). Logistics indicators assessment tool. Arlington, VA, John Snow International .

Diallo K et al. (2003). Monitoring and evaluation of human resources for health: an international perspective. *Human Resources for Health*, 1:3.

Diaz-Monsalve SJ (2003). Measuring the job performance of district health managers in Latin America. *Annals of Tropical Medicine and Parasitology*, 97:299–311.

Diaz-Monsalve SJ (2004). The impact of health-management training programs in Latin America on job performance. *Cad Saude Publica*, 20:1110–1120.

Dieleman M et al. (2003). Identifying factors for job motivation of rural health workers in North Viet Nam. *Human Resources for Health*, 1:10.

Dolmans D, Schmidt H (1996). The advantages of problem-based curricula. *Postgraduate Medical Journal*, 72:535-538.

Dovlo D (1999). Report on issues affecting the mobility and retention of health workers in Commonwealth African States. Unpublished report to Commonwealth Secretariat, Arusha Tanzania

Dreesch N et al. (2005). An approach to estimating human resource requirements to achieve the Millennium Development Goals. *Health Policy and Planning*, 20:267–276.

Egger D et al. (2000). *Achieving the right balance: the role of policymaking processes in managing human resources for health problems – issues in health services delivery*. Geneva, World Health Organization.

English M et al. (2004). Assessment of inpatient paediatric care in first referral level hospitals in 13 districts in Kenya. *Lancet*, 363:1948–1953.

Ensor T, Duran-Moreno A (2002). Corruption as a challenge to effective regulation in the health sector. In: Saltman R, Busse R, Mossialos E, eds. *Regulating entrepreneurial behaviour in European health care systems*. Philadelphia, Open University Press.

Ferlie E, Shortell S (2001). Improving the quality of health care in the United Kingdom and the United States: a framework for change. *Milbank Quarterly*, 79:281–315.

Ferrinho P, Lerberghe WV, eds (2000). *Providing health care under adverse conditions: health personnel performance and individual coping strategies*. Antwerp, Belgium, ITG Press (Studies in Health Services Organisation and Policy).

Ferrinho P et al. (1998). How and why public sector doctors engage in private practice in Portuguese-speaking African countries. *Health Policy and Planning*, 13:332–338.

Font F et al. (2002). Paediatric referrals in rural Tanzania: the Kilombero District Study – a case series. *BMC International Health and Human Rights*, 2:4.

Forcier MB et al. (2004). Impact, regulation and health policy implications of physician migration in OECD countries. *Human Resources for Health*, 2:12.

Fort AL, Voltero L (2004). Factors affecting the performance of maternal health care providers in Armenia. *Human Resources for Health* , 2:8.

Franco LM et al. (2002). Health sector reform and public sector health worker motivation: a conceptual framework. *Social Science and Medicine*, 54:1255–1266.

Franco LM et al. (2004). Determinants and consequences of health worker motivation in hospitals in Jordan and Georgia. *Social Science and Medicine*, 58:343–355.

Frank B (2005). Commentary to 'Quality in graduate nursing education by William Holzemer'. *Nursing education perspectives*, 26:238–243.

Ghana Ministry of Health (2000). *Consolidating the gains, managing the challenges: 1999 health sector review*. Accra, Ghana, Ministry of Health.

Gladwin J et al. (2002). Rejection of an innovation: health information management training materials in east Africa. *Health Policy and Planning*, 17:354–361.

Goni S (1999). An analysis of the effectiveness of Spanish primary health care teams. *Health Policy*, 48:107–117.

Gould-Williams J (2004). The effects of 'high commitment' HRM practices on employee attitude: the views of public sector workers. *Public Administration*, 82:63–81.

Gray AM et al. (1996). The costs of nursing turnover: evidence from the British National Health Service. *Health Policy*, 38:117–128.

Green A, Collins C (2003). Health systems in developing countries: public sector managers and the management of contradictions and change. *The International Journal of Health Planning and Management*, 18(Suppl. 1):S67–S78.

Greenfield S et al. (1985). Expanding patient involvement in care: effects on patient outcomes. *Annals of Internal Medicine*, 102:520–528.

Gruen R et al. (2002). Dual job holding practitioners in Bangladesh: an exploration. *Social Science and Medicine*, 54:267–279.

Gupta N et al. (2003). Uses of population census data for monitoring geographical imbalance in the health workforce: snapshots from three developing countries. *International Journal for Equity in Health*, 2:11.

Hall JA et al. (1988). Meta-analysis of correlates of provider behavior in medical encounters. *Medical Care*, 26:657–675.

Hall T (2001). HRH data: guidelines and data requirements for a human resources for health information system. Geneva, World Health Organization.

Hanson CM et al. (1990). Factors related to job satisfaction and autonomy as correlates of potential job retention for rural nurses. *Journal of Rural Health*, 6:302–316.

Harris J (1978). *Critical characteristics of an accreditable institution, basic purposes of accreditation, and nontraditional forms of most concern*. Washington, DC, Council on Postsecondary Accreditation Project to Develop Evaluative Criteria and Procedures for the Accreditation of Nontraditional Education (Research Reports No. 2.6l-IO5).

Hartley HJ, Kramer JA (1991). Time management and leadership styles: an empirical study of long-term health care administrators. *Journal of Health Administration Education*, 9:307–322.

Helfenbein S et al. (1987). *Technologies for management information systems in primary health care*. Geneva, World Federation of Public Health Agencies.

Henderson Betkus M, MacLeod ML (2004). Retaining public health nurses in rural British Columbia: the influence of job and community satisfaction. *Canadian Journal of Public Health*, 95:54–58.

Hersey P et al. (2001). *Management of organizational behavior: leading human resources*. Upper Saddle River, NJ, Prentice Hall.

Hesterly SC, Robinson M (1990). Alternative caregivers: cost-effective utilization of R.N.s. *Nursing Administration Quarterly*, 14:18–23.

Hornby P, Forte P (2000). *Human resource indicators to monitor health service performance*. Geneva, World Health Organization.

Huber DL et al. (2000). Evaluating nursing administration instruments. *Journal of Nursing Administration*, 30:251–272.

Huber M, Orosz E (2003). Health expenditure trends in OECD countries, 1990-2001. *Health care financing review*, 25:1–22.

Huddart J, Picazo O (2003). *The health sector human resource crisis in Africa: an issues paper*. Washington, DC, SARA Project, Academy for Educational Development, USAID.

Humphreys J et al. (2001). A critical review of rural medical workforce retention in Australia. *Australian Health Review*, 24:91–102.

ILO (1998). *Terms of employment and working conditions in health sector reforms*. Geneva, International Labour Office.

Jackson J et al. (2003). A comparative assessment of West Virginia's financial incentive programs for rural physicians. *J Rural Health*, 19 (Suppl.):329–339.

Johns GH et al. (2001). Career retention in the dental hygiene workforce in Texas. *Journal of Dental Hygiene*, 75:135–148.

Joint Learning Initiative (2004). *Human resources for health*. Boston, MA, Harvard University Press.

Juhl N et al. (1993). Job satisfaction of rural public and home health nurses. *Public Health Nursing*, 10:42–47.

Junious DL et al. (2004). A study of school nurse job satisfaction. *Journal of School Nursing*, 20:88–93.

Kaplan SH et al. (1989). Assessing the effects of physician–patient interactions on the outcomes of chronic disease. *Medical Care*, 27(Suppl.):S110–S127.

Kaplan SH et al. (1995). Patient and visit characteristics related to physicians' participatory decision-making style. Results from the Medical Outcomes Study. *Medical Care*, 33:1176–1187.

Kaufman A et al. (1989). The New Mexico experiment: educational innovation and institutional change. *Academic Medicine*, 64:285–294.

Kenya Ministry of Health and Partnerships for Health Reform (1999). *Kenya National Health Accounts 1994*. Bethesda, MD, Partnerships for Health Reform, Abt Associates Inc.

Kersten J et al. (1991). Motivating factors in a student's choice of nursing as a career. *Journal of Nursing Education*, 30:30–33.

Kinnersley P et al. (2000). Randomised controlled trial of nurse practitioner versus general practitioner care for patients requesting "same day" consultations in primary care. *British Medical Journal*, 320:1043–1048.

Klitgaard R (2000). Subverting corruption. *Finance and Development*, 37(2):2-5.

Koh H Goh C (1995). An analysis of the factors affecting the turnover intention of non-managerial clerical staff: a Singapore study. *International Journal of Human Resource Management*, 6:103–125.

Kolehmainen-Aitken R-L (1992). The impact of decentralization on health workforce development in Papua New Guinea. *Public Administration and Development*, 12:175–191.

Kolehmainen-Aitken RL (2004). Decentralization's impact on the health workforce: perspectives of managers, workers and national leaders. *Human Resources for Health*, 2:5.

Kruseman A et al. (1997). Problem-based learning at Maastricht: an assessment of cost and outcome. *Education for Health*, 10:179–187.

Larsen PD et al. (2003). Factors influencing career decisions: perspectives of nursing students in three types of programs. *Journal of Nursing Education*, 42:168–173.

Lawrence J, Greene K (1980). *A question of quality: the higher education ratings game*. Washington DC: AAHE-ERIC (Higher Education Research Report No. 5).

Lee SH et al. (1991). Job and life satisfaction among rural public health nurses in Taiwan. *Asia-Pacific Journal of Public Health*, 5:331–338.

Lerberghe WV et al. (2000). Performance, working conditions and coping strategies: an introduction. In: Ferrinho P, Lerberghe WV eds. *Providing health care under adverse conditions: health personnel performance and individual coping strategies*. Antwerp, Belgium, ITG Press.

Lin Y, Tavrow P (2000). *Assessing health worker performance of IMCI in Kenya. Quality assurance project case study*. Bethesda, MD, Quality Assurance Project.

Lippeveld T et al. (2000). *Design and implementation of health information systems*. Geneva, World Health Organization.

Mackereth P (1989). An investigation of the developmental influences on nurses' motivation for their continuing education. *Journal of Advanced Nursing*, 14:776–787.

Majoor G (2004). Recent innovations in education of human resources for health. Joint Learning Initiative (JLI) Working paper 2-3, draft version.

Malawi Ministry of Health and Population, and Department of Planning (2001). *Malawi National Health Accounts (NHA): a broader perspective of the Malawian health sector*. Lilongwe, Malawi: Ministry of Health and Population..

Marchal B Kegels G (2003). Health workforce imbalances in times of globalization: brain drain or professional mobility? *International Journal of Health Planning and Management*, 18(Suppl. 1):S89–S101.

Martineau T, Martinez J (1997). *Human resources in the health sector: guidelines for appraisal and strategic development*. Brussels, European Commission.

Martinez J, Martineau T (1998). Rethinking human resources: an agenda for the millennium. *Health Policy and Planning*, 13:345–358.

Meterko M et al. (2004). Teamwork culture and patient satisfaction in hospitals. *Medical Care*, 42:492–498.

MSH (1998). *Human resource development (HRD) assessment instrument for non-governmental organizations (NGOs) and public sector health organizations*. Cambridge, MA: Management Sciences for Health.

Munro BH (1983). Job satisfaction among recent graduates of schools of nursing. *Nursing Research*, 32:350–355.

Murillo MV (undated). *Latin American unions and the reform of social service delivery systems: institutional constraints and policy change*. Washington, DC, Inter-American Development Bank.

Mutziwa-Mangiza D (1998). *The impact of health sector reform on public sector health worker motivation in Zimbabwe*. Bethesda, MD, Abt Associates, Partnerships for Health Reform.

Nandakumar AK et al. (2004). *Synthesis of findings from NHA studies in twenty-six countries*. Bethesda, MD, Abt Associates.

Ndumbe PM (2003). *The training of human resources for health in Africa*. Joint Learning Initiative on Human Resources for Health, Rockefeller Foundation, Africa Working Group. Available online at http://www.globalhealthtrust.org/doc/abstracts/WG4/NdumbeHRHFINAL.pdf.

Newbrander W, Thomason J (1988). Computerising a national health system in Papua New Guinea. *Health Policy and Planning*, 3:255–259.

Nordberg E et al. (1996). Exploring the interface between first and second level of care: referrals in rural Africa. *Tropical Medicine and International Health*, 1:107–111.

Ohara K et al. (1998). Study of a patient referral system in the Republic of Honduras. *Health Policy and Planning*, 13:433–445.

Padarath A et al. (2003). *Health personnel in Southern Africa: confronting maldistribution and brain drain*. Regional Network for Equity in Health in Southern Africa (EQUINET), Health Systems Trust (South Africa), MEDACT (United Kingdom). Available online at http://www.equinetafrica.org/policy.html.

PAHO (2001). *Report on the Technical Meeting on Managed Migration of Skilled Nursing Personnel*. Bridgetown, Barbados, Pan American Health Organization, Caribbean Office.

Parker C Rickman B (1995). Economic determinants of the labor force withdrawal of registered nurses. *Journal of Economics and Finance*, 19:17–26.

Pong RW et al. (1995). *Health human resources in community-based health care: a review of the literature*. Health Canada, Health Promotion and Programs Branch. Available online at http://www.hc-sc.gc.ca/hcs-sss/pubs/care-soins/1995-build-plan-commun/build-plan-commun1/index_e.html.

Pugno PA, McPherson DS (2002). The role of international medical graduates in family practice residencies. *Family Medicine*, 34:468–469.

Raja S et al. (2000). *Uganda logistics systems for public health commodities: an assessment report*. Washington, DC, USAID.

Razali SM (1996). Medical school entrance and career plans of Malaysian medical students. *Medical Education*, 30:418–423.

Reich MR (1996). Applied political analysis for health reform. *Current Issues in Public Health*, 2:186–191.

Roberts MJ (2004). *Getting health reform right: a guide to improving performance and equity*. New York, Oxford University Press.

Roenen C et al. (1997). How African doctors make ends meet: an exploration. *Tropical Medicine and International Health*, 2:127–135.

Rondeau KV Wagar TH (2001). Impact of human resource management practices on nursing home performance. *Health Services Management Research*, 14:192–202.

Rose-Ackerman S (1997). The political economy of corruption. In: Elliot K ed. *Corruption and the global economy*. Washington, DC, Institute for International Economics.

Roter D et al. (1991). Sex differences in patients' and physicians' communication during primary care medical visits. *Medical Care*, 29:1083–1093.

Ruck NF et al. (1999). Assessing management training needs: a study in the Punjab health services, Pakistan. *Journal of Health and Population in Developing Countries*, 2:78–87.

Saltman RB, Von Otter C (1995). *Implementing planned markets in health care: balancing social and economic responsibility*. Buckingham, Open University Press.

Sandiford P et al. (1992). What can information systems do for primary health care? An international perspective. *Social Science and Medicine*, 34:1077–1087.

Sararaks S, Jamaluddin R (1999). Demotivating factors among government doctors in Negeri Sembilan. *Medical Journal of Malaysia*, 54:310–319.

Schlette S (1998). *Public service reforms and their impact on health sector personnel in Colombia*. Geneva, World Health Organization.

Scott T et al. (2003a). The quantitative measurement of organizational culture in health care: a review of the available instruments. *Health Services Research*, 38:923–945.

Scott T et al. (2003b). Does organisational culture influence health care performance? A review of the evidence. *Journal of Health Services Research and Policy*, 8:105–117.

Shah MA et al. (2001). Determinants of job satisfaction among selected care providers in Kuwait. *Journal of Allied Health*, 30:68–74.

Shortell SM et al. (1991). Organizational assessment in intensive care units (ICUs): construct development, reliability, and validity of the ICU nurse-physician questionnaire. *Medical Care*, 29:709–726.

Shortell SM et al. (1994). The performance of intensive care units: does good management make a difference? *Medical Care*, 32:508–525.

Shum C et al. (2000). Nurse management of patients with minor illnesses in general practice: multicentre, randomised controlled trial. *British Medical Journal*, 320:1038–1043.

Siddiqi S et al. (2001). The effectiveness of patient referral in Pakistan. *Health Policy and Planning*, 16:193–198.

Simoes EA et al. (2003). Management of severely ill children at first-level health facilities in sub-Saharan Africa when referral is difficult. *Bulletin of the World Health Organization*, 81:522–531.

Siziya S Woelk G (1995). Predictive factors for medical students and housemen to work in rural health institutions in Zimbabwe. *Cent Afr J Med*, 41:252–254.

Stevens KA Walker EA (1993). Choosing a career: why not nursing for more high school seniors? *Journal of Nursing Education*, 32:13–37.

Stilwell B et al. (2003). Developing evidence-based ethical policies on the migration of health workers: conceptual and practical challenges. *Human Resources for Health*, 1:8.

Stordeur S et al. (2001). Leadership, organizational stress, and emotional exhaustion among hospital nursing staff. *Journal of Advanced Nursing*, 35:533–542.

Tawfik L, Kinoti SN (2003). *The impact of HIV/AIDS on the health workforce in sub-Saharan Africa*. Washington, DC, Support for Analysis and Research in Africa Project (SARA), USAID.

Tawfik, L., Kinoti, S. (2006) The impact of HIV/AIDS on the health workforce in developing countries. Background paper prepared for The world health report 2006 – working together for health. http://www.who.int/hrh/documents/Impact_of_HIV.pdf

Tri DL (1991). The relationship between primary health care practitioners' job satisfaction and characteristics of their practice settings. *Nurse Practitioner*, 16:46, 49–52, 55.

Troutt WE (1979). Regional accreditation, evaluation criteria, and quality assurance. *Journal of Higher Education*, 50:199–210.

Tzeng HM (2002). The influence of nurses' working motivation and job satisfaction on intention to quit: an empirical investigation in Taiwan. *International Journal of Nursing Studies*, 39:867–878.

Van Lerberghe W et al. (2002a). Human resources impact assessment. *Bulletin of the World Health Organization*, 80:525.

Van Lerberghe W et al. (2002b). When staff is underpaid: dealing with the individual coping strategies of health personnel. *Bulletin of the World Health Organization*, 80: 581–584.

Vandenberghe C (1999). Organizational culture, person–culture fit, and turnover: a replication in the health care industry. *Journal of Organizational Behavior*, 20:175–184.

Venning P et al. (2000). Randomised controlled trial comparing cost effectiveness of general practitioners and nurse practitioners in primary care. *British Medical Journal*, 320:1048–1053.

Verbrugge LM Steiner RP (1981). Physician treatment of men and women patients: sex bias or appropriate care? *Medical Care*, 19:609–632.

Villeneuve MJ (1994). Recruiting and retaining men in nursing: a review of the literature. *Journal of Professional Nursing*, 10:217–228.

Vujicic M et al. (2004). The role of wages in the migration of health care professionals from developing countries. *Human Resources for Health*, 2:3.

Wahba J (2003). *Health labor markets: incentives or institutions?* UK: University of Southampton. Working Group 7, Joint Learning Initiative on Human Resources for Health and Development. Global Health Trust, Harvard University.

Waldman JD et al. (2004). The shocking cost of turnover in health care. *Health Care Management Review*, 29:2–7.

Wibulpolprasert S, Pengpaibon P (2003). Integrated strategies to tackle the inequitable distribution of doctors in Thailand: four decades of experience. *Human Resources for Health*, 1:12.

World Bank (1993). *Investing in health*. New York, Oxford University Press.

World Bank (1994a). *Adjustment in Africa: reforms, results, and the road ahead*. New York: Oxford University Press.

World Bank (1994b). *Better health in Africa: experience and lessons learned*. Washington, DC, World Bank.

World Bank (2003). *Assessment tool for human resources management records and information systems*. World Bank. Available online at http://www1.worldbank.org/publicsector/civilservice/acrext/assessmenttool.pdf.

World Bank (2004). *World development indicators*. Washington DC: World Bank.

WFME (2003). *Basic medical education: WFME global standards for quality improvement*. Copenhagen, World Federation for Medical Education.

WHO (2000). *The world health report 2000 – health systems: improving performance*. Geneva, World Health Organization.

WHO (2001). *WHO guidelines for quality assurance of basic medical education in the Western Pacific Region*. Manila, Philippines.

WHO (2002). *Human resources and national health systems: final report*. Geneva, World Health Organization.

WHO (2003a). *The world health report 2003 – shaping the future*. Geneva, World Health Organization.

WHO (2003b). *Migration of health professionals in six countries: a synthesis report*. Brazzaville, WHO Regional Office for Africa.

WHO (2004). *WHO estimates of health personnel: physicians, nurses, midwives, dentists, pharmacists*. Geneva, World Health Organization.

WHO (2006). *The world health report 2006 – working together for health*. Geneva, World Health Organization.

WHO and UNICEF (1978). *Declaration of Alma-Ata*. Alma Ata, USSR, World Health Organization: 79.

Yaktin US et al. (2003). Personal characteristics and job satisfaction among nurses in Lebanon. *Journal of Nursing Administration*, 33:384–390.

Yaping D, Stanton P (2002). Evaluation of the health services management training course of Jiangsu, China. *Australian Health Review Rev*, 25:161–170.

Zhou J Zhang X (1994). The causes and solutions of red envelopes in hospitals. *Chinese Journal of Hospital Administration*, 10:353–355.

Zimmerman JE et al. (1993). Improving intensive care: observations based on organizational case studies in nine intensive care units: a prospective, multicenter study. *Critical Care Medicine*, 21(10):1443–1451.

Zurn P et al. (2002). *Imbalances in the health workforce: briefing paper*. Geneva, World Health Organization: 1–51.